Blue Eyes Love Red Roses

The Essential Ilene – Ruth Ilene Lindquist

Blue Eyes
Love Red Roses

The Essential Ilene – Ruth Ilene Lindquist

By Oiva Herbert Lindquist

Blue Eyes Love Red Roses
The Essential Ilene – Ruth Ilene Lindquist

The title of this book and the photo on the front cover are related to the poem on page 75.

Printed in the United States of America.
First edition.

ISBN-13: 978-1537092294
ISBN-10: 1537092294

Produced by Smiling Dog Design

Foreward

Your beauty is that of your inner self, the unfolding beauty of a gentle and quiet spirit, which is of great value in God's sight.
1 Peter 3:4

Ruth Ilene joyfully believed in a risen Jesus Christ. She was an energetic, attractive young woman with large, blue smiling eyes. The eyes reflected a friendly, gregarious person who realistically participated in and enjoyed life. She was without pretense or subterfuge while lovingly interacting with her destiny.

Ilene was severely handicapped by polio in September 1952. This was equivalent to a bomb landing in the middle of our happy family. This book is the record of her struggles to victory and triumph until her death in 2007.

You will read about a courageous woman's interaction with life despite her limitations and problems. She did not avoid facts or problems.

Ilene's heritage was Scotch, English and Irish. Her mother's Purcell family Scotch ancestry contributed tenacity. The Irish came from the Bechtels. She was, as the song says:

> *When Irish eyes are smiling,*
> *Sure, tis like a morn in spring.*
> *In the lilt of Irish laughter*
> *You can hear the angels sing,.*
> *When Irish hearts are happy,*
> *All the world seems bright and gay.*
> *And when Irish eyes are smiling,*
> *Sure, they steal your heart away.*

Ilene spent a great deal of time and thought in giving her annual talk to the members of the Stephen Ministry of Woodlake Lutheran Church in Richfield, Minnesota. The Stephen Ministry was a visitation program to homebound. This was a unique speech by an individual who considered this ministry a major element in their life. She considered this speech a mission of her life.

The words Ilene spoke were totally her own and she worked hard to make them personal and relevant. Her speech, which is at the end of this book, was a culmination of years of effort first started by a request from the Reverend Robert Hall of our church.

Ilene's address was well received by the group and was an inspiration to many of them. A physically handicapped woman in a wheelchair, with a loving, accepting spirit who obviously enjoyed life and worshiped God was an impelling speaker. She wanted to contribute to someone else. This was exactly the thrust of the Stephen's Ministry program.

This book was written to help understand the "Essential Ilene," a Christian woman of great courage and love for family and of great faith and love for her Lord and Savior Jesus Christ. Proceeds from the sale of this book will be donated to a scholarship in Ilene's name at Augsburg College in Minneapolis, Minnesota, for women who are studying physics.

Table of Contents

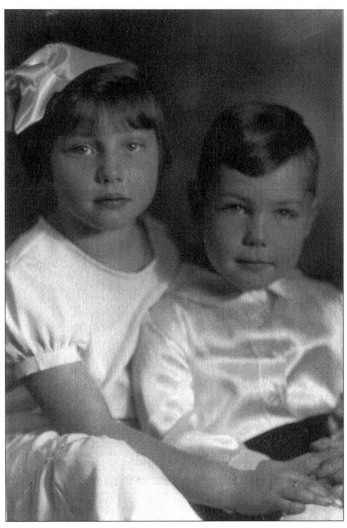

Ruth Ilene and brother Dave.

CHAPTER 1

Before the Polio Bomb

The meaning and basis for actions in our own history need to include the events and starting point of our story. In Ilene's case, it is especially important. Before Ilene wrote the "First Note" to me, she had an active physical life, including a caring Christian home, four years of a loving full marriage and a faith in a risen Jesus Christ.

Ilene was connected to the real world and the enjoyment of life. Her father Harold was a "good feeler" who enjoyed his horticultural work and gardening, weekly square dances, friends and his family. Ilene was a replica of Harold; she fully enjoyed life and was interested in doing many things. She was also clearly the daughter of her mother Blanche, a trained nurse. Ilene was also strong, courageous and dedicated to the care of others. During her college years, she had been in a Navy nursing program at the University of Iowa. She left the program when WWII ended.

Ilene had a personal daily devotion in which she brought the names of her family members and those she loved to God in prayer. Ilene knew she was a person known personally to God, and she had a mission in life. The devotion was a private inward pilgrimage with God.

The Bechtel home was on Arbor Street, just three blocks from the Iowa State University campus in Ames, Iowa. Ilene would, as a little girl, wander on the campus and visit places such as the White Swans on Lake Lagoon, the horse barns, the Campanile (a memorial bell tower) and the workshop of Christian Peterson, the Iowa State University sculpture artist.

There was an openness in Ilene's demeanor that stated that she wanted you to know her. As a child, she always sought new playmates and got acquainted with newcomers to her Arbor Street neighborhood. Some of these playmates became lifelong friends such as Alice Jean Miller and Hazel Norton. Ilene's father Harold joined in her neighborliness by calling Alice Jean "Sweet Alice." She and Ilene played tennis, joined Girl Scouts and had the long conversations of normal young girls.

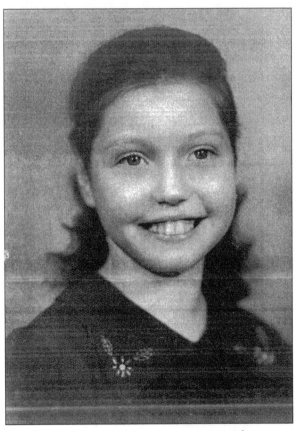

The "Essential Ilene" as a young girl.

Ilene helped to organize and energetically participated in the neighborhood "Olympic Games" which included boys. In competition, she was physically gifted and held her ground against all comers. She possessed and developed as a child the strength of character and winsome personal qualities that would remain with her all her life.

The Collegiate Presbyterian Church of Ames was three blocks from Ilene's house and was an integral part of her life as she was growing up. Dr. Barlow, a dour Scot, was the pastor of the church that included many college members. Ilene's parents were active in the church. Harold served in many roles from elder to being a bath-robed wise man in the annual Christmas program. Mother Blanche worked in the congregation in many roles from decorating the church to kitchen duties. She fussed about "professors' wives" being reluctant to do their share. Ilene was required to do memory work, which stayed with her for life. She knew all the books of the Bible and many verses from scripture, and she had a faith in God.

The Bechtel family was from a Paunee, Nebraska, farm and moved to Ames so that Ilene and her brother Dave would have the opportunity to attend Iowa State University. Ilene was a 1949 Zoology major. Her brother Dave graduated later and became a leader in Iowa's public school system.

Ilene and I met at a Friday night college "mixer" at the Iowa State University student union, the main social center of the college. I was in the Navy V-12 program at the college. I arrived after some other activities. Ilene came after finishing her job at Ma Tilden's candy store. I picked out the prettiest girl in the ballroom. She was a tall girl who was wearing an orange, red and tan-plaid dress. We started dancing and enjoying life. She was without pretenses or guile and was a great dancer. I enjoyed being with her.

3

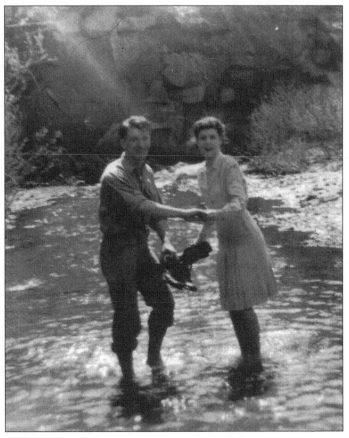

Joy – wading in Ledges Park, Boone, Iowa.

A short time later I was given two tickets to the college Count Basie dance for working on the physics department's annual, week-long VEISHA open house. Since Ilene and I had just become acquainted at about that time, I had intended to ask Ilene to the dance but had not done so. I found out at a later time that Ilene's father was miffed with me, as was Ilene, for not having done so. Count Basie and his band in person was a major experience.

His swing music and way of playing were conducive to a fun night. He had a way of orchestrating the band with his piano that was punctuation and structure. The Count had a smooth-jazz approach with great punch from the horns. His band was very much suited to the style of dancing that we enjoyed. Ilene and I attended the event and had a very memorable time.

One of our first dates was a visit to Ledges Park in Boone, about 15 miles west of Ames. Ilene asked if I had ever gone wading in a creek. We happily waded into the stream and were photographed by my Navy pal, Don Wilson.

Pete Lundquist of Honeywell later made a painting for us from this photo. The painting captured this wonderful and meaningful moment in our life. The painting is currently a feature in our living room in our house in Richfield.

Our relationship progressed and we began dating regularly. We attended the Ames Bethesda Lutheran Church on Sundays and the inter-varsity Christian Fellowship during the week.

We had a Navy open house at Friley Hall to which I invited Ilene. I had an attractive photo of Elaine, my high school girl-friend, on my desk. Subsequently I received a new, very attractive photo to add to my desk "from my buddy." At that time, Ilene and I were friends or buddies.

When I was discharged from the Navy, Ilene suggested that I live at Mrs. Battel's home on Arbor Street. It was cozy and in a very convenient location since it was next door to the Bechtel's home. Ilene managed to greet me after classes. She was a warm, "Essential Ilene"

Later I invited Ilene to my home in Cloquet, Minnesota, during the Christmas vacation. She had been visiting her aunt Grace Pulver in Minneapolis. We visited Duluth and its curling club where we saw our first hockey game together – the Duluth Coleratures versus the Canadian Fort Frances' team.

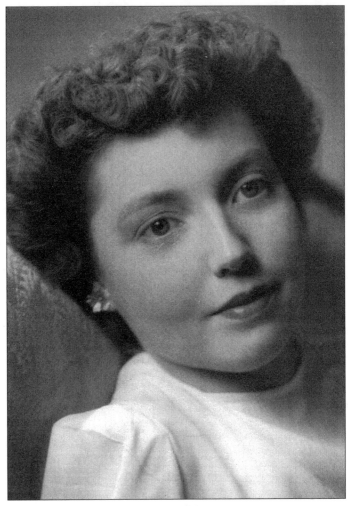

My "Buddy."

It was a below-zero December night in an unheated arena. The intermissions emptied the hockey arena with everyone scrambling for coffee or hot chocolate. The goalie for the winning Coleratures was Frank Brimcheck, a big man who had played

NHL hockey for the Chicago Black Hawks. The memory of our first hockey game was an especially fond one for us. This experience seemed to foreshadow the many cold winters' nights that we spent watching our grandson Eric's hockey games. Sometime later, Ilene and I again rendézvoused at Christmas in Cloquet at my parent's home. We also stopped by Savolian's Jewelry (a Finnish jeweler) in Duluth to admire wedding rings. I later purchased a ring for our engagement. The wedding took place on June 11, 1948, and was a joyous event. My parents drove down from Cloquet to Ames and enjoyed themselves, thanks to the hospitality of Ilene's parents.

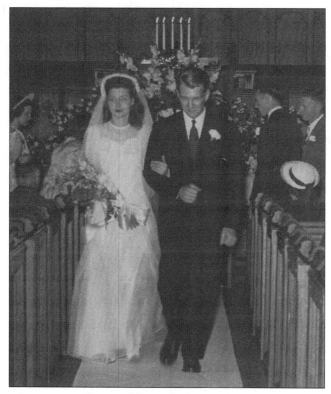

Our wedding – June 11, 1948.

We honeymooned for a month – two weeks at Harry Pulver's cabin on Gull Lake courtesy of Ilene's Aunt Grace, and spent an additional two weeks touring in our 1928 Willys-Knight touring coupe. We purchased the rumble- seated car from a lady who had never driven during the winter, keeping the car stored up on blocks. The car was amazing in that it drove silently. It had a sleeve-valve engine that eliminated all valve popping. It is now listed as a classic car, but my father felt it was a most impractical car that no one could repair.

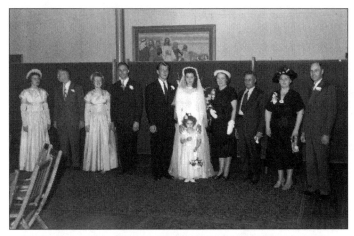

Wedding party – basement of the Collegiate Presbyterian Church, Ames, Iowa.

Our touring of northern Minnesota and nearby Canada was by tent and ignorance. I had studied tourist propaganda and found the Boundary Waters Canoe Area Wilderness. Ilene retained her composure and still insisted on boiling any water we used. She was a scientist and nurse.

We then stayed with my folks in Cloquet until school started in the fall. My father worked at the Northwest Paper Company, my mother at Diamond Match Company. I worked at the Weyerhaeuser Company warehouse in the shipping department. I was part of a crew that loaded railroad boxcars with Weyerhaeuser's housing products. Ilene failed to get a job at the "prestigious" mill. Instead, she managed the household. I was a most admired worker since I had such an attractive lady pick me up after work.

Ed Wicklund, our next-door neighbor who was on the same crew at the Weyerhaeuser plant as I was, told me I didn't understand work at the mill as it took 28 years on the same job to get the real meaning of the job (i.e., the hopelessness of the situation). He also felt Ilene and I saw the world through some type of love glasses.

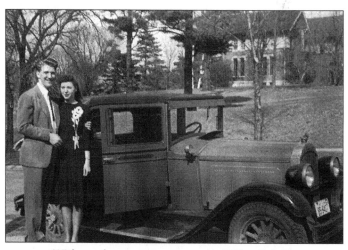

With our honeymoon car – the Willys Knight

Prior to leaving for school, we advertised in the Cloquet Pine Journal to sell the Willys. My father was sure no one would want to buy the car. Ilene sold the car to a local resident for $250 more than we paid for it. A second buyer came by who offered to more than match the first offer. Ilene declined.

When I first met Ilene, I wondered if she could fit into a Finnish community of saunas, polka dancing and with my immigrant parents. My mother had attended grade school in Wisconsin but my father had never been to any school and spoke English poorly. Their immigrant background could have been difficult for a wife to accept. But Ilene enjoyed the challenge, as later evidenced by 4th of July at the Brule River Co-op Hall.

It was the tradition in the immigrant Finnish community to celebrate holidays with celebrations at established dance halls. One such hall was the Brule River Co-op Hall in Wisconsin. It was one of the premium locations for "Juhlas" – high festivities.

In the second summer after our marriage, my parents found out that Viola Turpinen and her orchestra were at the Brule River dance hall for the weekend. Viola was the best Finnish-American accordion player for the Finnish community. She lived in New York in the Finnish community of the Bronx, a part of the Finnish labor movement. She had been born in the USA but was everywhere regarded as the "Finnish Princess." She was well known in America and played in Finland.

Viola's summers were spent in touring the Midwest as the premier accordion player in America. Her big, pearl-studded accordion that was proudly labeled "Viola" produced the music for joyful dancers who flocked to her dances. It was a special night to have her play at the 4th of July celebration in Brule. The schottisches, polkas and yenkas (a Finnish folk dance) were played in a lively beat with a great deal of intricate fingering adding to the melody of the compositions. This was the best; the event of each year.

My father took Ilene and me to this dance with a great deal of pleasure. Despite being a very hot day in July, he was dressed in his best three-piece brown-wool suit of good quality. My mother was in her best blue dress and was very proud to be the mother of her son and daughter-in-law. For our family, it was a great highlight to be there amongst the observing Finnish community.

My father loved to dance this type of music and had had a lot of experience doing it. It was obviously a moment of great pleasure for my mother to dance with me at the Brule Hall to the music of Viola.

Ilene enjoyed Scandinavian dancing. She had taken a course in Scandinavian dancing and was with her parents at many of the folk dances at Iowa State University. She was especially good at following her partner's lead. The dancers were all accustomed to moving in a circle around the dance floor.

From my vantage point, the Finnish Princess Viola was especially lively in the melody and beat of the yenka. I did not know how to dance a yenka; my father seemed to be an expert.

My father and Ilene danced by me and created a memory for me of my smiling, happy father whose brown-toed shoes seemed to twinkle with every beat and note that Viola played. My father was hot and had unbuttoned his coat. His wavy hair was moist and down on his brow, but I saw that he was in one of the most joyful moments of his life. Ilene was following his every lead and was laughing as she moved with ease to his every direction and pause. She had dressed for the hot weather in a flowing, yellow-plaid cotton dress that permitted air movement. As the two synchronized dancers moved by me that night, they left me with an emotion-packed memory. I have the vivid, meaningful memory of my happy father who could really dance, and a vivid memory of the feelings of pride that I felt that my tall, attractive bride had been more than equal to the task of dancing with my Finnish father.

Ilene could pass any test or situation in my family relationships. She could walk to the remote blueberry patches of the Corona Swamp amidst an onslaught of mosquitoes. She could enjoy the Finnish sauna in my father's basement and enjoy meeting my country relatives. She was a "real" person who could adapt to any situation.

We lived in Ames one year after our marriage while Ilene obtained a degree in zoology. I obtained a master's degree in education. I concentrated on a minor in physics to fill in some areas such as statistics, and tests and measurements. The courses in statistics and measurements later proved invaluable. I taught physics laboratory courses to supplement my GI-Bill income.

Our good friends, the Borgendales, suggested that we contact Augsburg College in Minneapolis for a position in physics. Arlene Borgendale had graduated from Augsburg and felt there might be a job there. This began a relationship with Augsburg that has continued to this day.

Teaching physics at Augsburg in a friendly Christian community was most enjoyable. Augsburg was a Lutheran Free Church College. At the time, Augsburg was a conservative school. Dancing was not an approved activity, but we felt it was a minor limitation.

Dr. Bernhard Christensen was the president of the college when we joined Augsburg. He was a man of great intellectual and spiritual life that he communicated to me. He wrote regarding the basic meaning of Christian education at Augsburg: "Much of the content of a Christian college education is not at all unique. But in spirit and approach, it is different. It approaches all the problems and realities of life in the spirit of prayer and faith. It reckons with the Power of God. Christian education is education sought in the conscious presence of God. It is education that reckons realistically with His power."

The years at Augsburg under Dr. Christensen and the opportunity to start a new curriculum were exciting to us. I was the first full-time physics teacher the college had ever had. Dr. Christensen's concept of Christian education began to be real to me.

We began to have visions of developing a biophysics curriculum that could partner with the nearby medical facilities at the University of Minnesota which were only blocks away. Ilene and I shared this "dream" since she was a science major who was interested in Medicine. I had just received my M.S. in biophysics at the University of Minnesota from Dr. Otto Schmitt. I had enrolled in Dr. Schmitt's Ph.D. biophysics program and he gave me a summer job in his facility. I enjoyed the studies in my program and now had some specific reasons to develop professionally. I had the feeling of one who had been "called."

Several of my students were outstanding, Ph.D.-caliber students and could form the basis for some strong research teams. Dr. Schmitt and Dr. Burr Steinbach of the physiology department at the U of M were well known scientists and could provide the basis for cooperation with Augsburg. They were friendly to me and encouraged me in obtaining a Ph.D. in biophysics. That vision included supplementing my Augsburg salary from research grants.

In addition to enjoying my work, Ilene and I had begun developing some friendships at Augsburg and at Trinity Lutheran Church that expanded the dimensions to our lives. Old Trinity Church was adjacent to the school and attended by many of the faculty. Pastor Martin Olson had us take confirmation together. Ilene had to be confirmed as a Lutheran in order to join Trinity. Ilene was in the class to understand Lutheranism and I was there to make up for my "suspect" confirmation in the Finnish Congregational Church. Ilene sang in the choir and became a member of the Sunshine Circle. This was the most spiritual-yet-cordial group of women Ilene had ever known.

Ilene was a winsome young lady whose charm and friendliness brought us many friends. As a tall beauty with a warm, honest simplicity, a smile and a lack of guile, she won many friends. She had, without trying, a way of making people want to be friendly with her (e.g., the butcher, the janitor and the college president).

It seemed that the plot of our lives had been established and we were happily playing our parts in a joyous play. Ilene was the beautiful long-legged wife in love with a new professor at Augsburg College. He was pursuing a Ph.D. while enjoying teaching as the first full-time physics professor at the college.

We began a search for a home of our own that would be within our means. With the help of Olaf Rogne, the financial leader at Augsburg, and Dick Pautz, a Trinity Church member who was a real estate agent, we located a very economical home in south Minneapolis. The house was a bargain because it was small and located on a half lot. The trolley tracks were in front of the house. We were able to obtain a mortgage that we could handle by borrowing the down payment from our parents. One aspect of the house was that it was located near a small park and about three blocks from Christ Church Lutheran. The renowned Finnish-American, Eliel Saarinen, designed this famous church. It was built in 1949 when we were moving into our home. In 2009 it was designated as a national landmark. Ilene and I visited the church one Sunday and were greatly impressed by a sense of serenity.

The south-facing church was dominated by a large, simple cross at the front of the church that was bathed in a Sunday-morning light from a curved, white front surface. The church and our house still stand, seemingly unchanged in their setting today. The trolley tracks are gone.

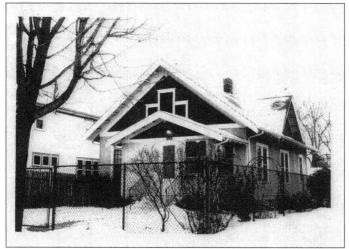

Our first home.

Our house by the trolley tracks was a totally happy place. We decorated the little house. A red-haired son, Martin Daniel ("Dan"), was born in July 1951. Dan's newly papered bedroom had a lively rose-colored collection of fun figures that surrounded his crib, a present from his loving Finnish grandparents. Each evening was a festive ceremony in which Daniel would jump gaily in the crib and repeat his joyful words "Beim, Beim, Beim," postponing going to sleep and completely filling his parents with happiness and love.

My study, a little bedroom, was transformed into Dan's nursery. I was trying to convert the old basement coal bin into my study. We were grateful to God for all our blessings and most aware of our personal happiness.

Ilene continued to decorate our new home. She painted the kitchen and breakfast nook in a warm green and papered the nook with a flowered paper with vines. The vines and the paint were a perfect match. The little nook off the kitchen was the cheeriest eating space we have ever had.

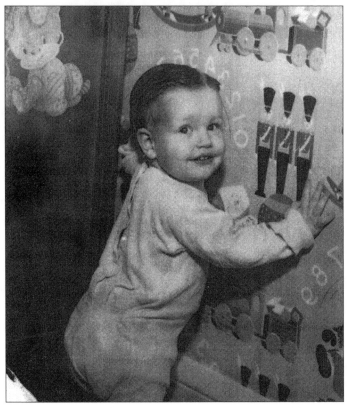

Dan – our "Beim-Beim" man who delayed going to sleep.

We papered the living room with a bold, square-design paper and found nothing was plum. We bought a remnant rug on sale from Montgomery Ward that we cut in half and re-sewed it to serve as our living room rug. We purchased a "Muntz" 17-inch TV.

We shared in the vision of having found our niche in life. Ilene was friendly to my students and hosted some of them at our little house. The wife of one of my students was apprehended stealing some money and the couple lost their apartment. Ilene invited them to live with us for a few days. Our small house was too small to support all of us, but we managed until they located a new place to live. The student later obtained a Ph.D. at the University of Minnesota and became a computer engineer at IBM.

We were grateful to God for all our blessings and most aware of our personal happiness. Our family had just been established and the future seemed secure. We felt God's blessing in our affairs. Our joyful lives were encompassed by our mutual faith in our Lord Jesus. We felt God's blessing in our affairs. We had a lovely surround for the anticipated arrival of our second child.

It was Labor Day weekend in Minneapolis. Ilene's parents from Ames, Iowa, were visiting with great-grandparents Estelle and Herb Bechtel. They all wanted to be near our precious baby boy who had captured everyone's love. Labor Day of 1952 was during a very hot week that included many days with temperatures in the 90s. The Minnesota State Fair was in progress. Ilene's folks were interested in comparing it to the Iowa State Fair.

The newspapers reported that the Stevenson versus Eisenhower presidential campaign was slow so far but that Eisenhower was headed by train for Minnesota on a "breakfast tour." The Yankees baseball team defeated the Washington Senators 6 to 1 with Mantle, Rizzuto, and Berra all getting hits. The Minneapolis Millers, a minor-league baseball team Ilene and I supported, were playing Ray Dandridge at third base and Billy Gardner on second.

Into this setting a dark cloud was looming of which we were unaware. The newspapers reported:

> *"The city reports 166 new polio cases for August,*
> *for a total of 201 cases, including nine deaths."*
> *The Sister Kenny Institute reported that it had*
> *20 staff therapists working around the clock*
> *in several hospitals.*

It was this setting into which a bombshell would explode in our own family.

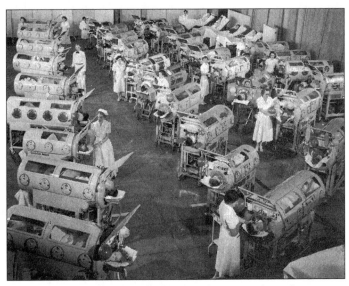

The iron lung enabled polio patients to breathe.

CHAPTER 2

The Battle to Survive

Little red-haired Dan knew something was wrong. He wandered around our little house, toddling as a plump, worried child. The 14-month-old went from his newly decorated front-bedroom nursery to our bedroom, checking on his beloved mommy who seemed very sick. He knew something was wrong and was trying to find out the problem that eluded his wordless search. He came to Mama's bedside and raised his hand for a moment and left quietly without answers to his concern. This was repeated a few minutes later.

On August 28, Ilene had a minor eye-focus problem at a drive-in movie. On August 29, she had a regular pregnancy check-up at Dr. Nesset's office. She reported backaches and headaches that aspirin didn't help. The doctor prescribed a sleeping medication from Keller Drug Store on Lake Street and Bloomington Avenue in south Minneapolis.

By Saturday, August 30, the drug had done nothing. I started taking Ilene's temperature, which was cycling up and down. I called Dr. Nesset with the information. The doctor came immediately to our house at 3425-38th Avenue in south Minneapolis. He examined Ilene and the temperature record I had taken. He began calling various hospitals for entrance for a polio case. He reluctantly concluded that Minneapolis General Hospital was the place for us to go and arranged for an examination.

He recommended that I take her there immediately. Ilene was still able to walk although she was weak. I took Ilene rapidly to General Hospital (now Hennepin County Medical Center) in our dark-green Plymouth coupe. The trip from our home to General

Hospital was lost in a blur. When we arrived at the hospital, I helped her in. Ilene was wearing a bright-blue satin slip as she weakly entered the examination room. What happened for 55 years after Ilene was admitted to Minneapolis General Hospital is the story that I must tell because it reveals a person of courage, faith and joy in the face of adversity.

As soon as we arrived, the nurses whisked Ilene away into isolation facilities for incoming polio victims. I was not allowed entrance to the polio ward and was separated from her. After completing some entrance forms, I was told to go home and they would call me with respect to her condition. They planned an immediate spinal tap, the key indicator for polio. Ilene was isolated in a small room where she quickly began to lose her physical capabilities.

After I left Ilene, she was alone with a disease that was rapidly sapping her of her capabilities. Since she was in a quarantined state, no one could visit and all communication ceased. She was told she could write a letter that would be delivered. I was not allowed to see her, but the first note was later given to me

A few hours later, the hospital called and requested that I come immediately to see Ilene and approve of some procedures that were needed. When I arrived, Ilene was obviously in a problematic condition. I kissed her as soon as I arrived, much to the chagrin of the nurses who were trying to maintain some quarantine conditions. Ilene assured me that the hospital was now going to take action to relieve her breathing problems and make things better. The procedures were a tracheotomy and the use of an iron lung. Once I had signed the form, I was told that I would be allowed to visit her when the procedures were accomplished.

From the isolation ward of Minneapolis General hospital, Ilene wrote a note to me in September 1952. The note was written to me at the onset of polio, praying for her return to taking care of her sons and me. She felt God had a purpose for her life despite whatever restrictions He had placed upon her.

NOTE 1

Dear Daddy,
I love you with all my heart.
You and our little sons are my life.
I long with all my being to be back
with you and take care of you.
Please pray to God that I have
the faith it takes to make me well
and strong.
   All my love,
   Fatty Ma

As can be seen, we had developed our personal name system in our relationship. She addressed me as "Daddy," a title from being the father of Dan and our unborn child. She was the complement of Daddy, "Fatty Ma." (Ilene had a tendency to gain weight during pregnancy). She expressed her love from her heart, an expression that was the depth of her being.

She expressed her desire to be back with our family and expressed her desire to be taking care of us. Her handwriting had disintegrated in this note but she requested prayer and the faith to be allowed to return.

When I next saw Ilene, she was in a stark, white hospital nightgown, alone in a small room. Her condition had deteriorated to the point that she seemed to be quickly going away. She was pleased to see me and began to assure me that once the procedures were completed she would be getting better. I was overwhelmed with the thought she was now concerned about me. I assured her that I would be standing by and available when she was done.

Ilene was five or six months pregnant when she was admitted to the hospital. The doctors hoped, as a minimum, she could carry the child two more weeks. There were four other mothers in the same condition as Ilene.

Three other cases were assembled into a larger room where they could be served better. Ilene was placed in a small hospital room by herself. All were under the care of Dr. James Bergquist, a young doctor who was very dedicated to caring for the eight lives in the four iron lungs.

It was a very hot fall in a non-air conditioned hospital. This presented additional problems. The cumbersome iron lung more than filled the small room. It was early history in providing breathing assistance.

In total, it was an overwhelming experience for the patient, their visitors and the attending nurses. The Brewster-Collins iron lung was not commodious to bodily functions that were needed. The odors in the room were sometimes similar to outdoor toilets on hot summer days. They might be tolerated for a short time, but overwhelming for hours. The hot weather problem was unusual for September, and reduced to tolerable in the fall. If forced to attend to a patient, nurses were very taxed. In one case, the nurse fainted while I was visiting Ilene, and I had to help her to leave the room. Other patients and families also surrounded us.

The image at night was awesome: One of the pumping of bellows at the end of the lung, portholes for viewing and access to the patient, and oxygen flowing to the tracheotomy in the patient's neck via heated-water chambers. In total, it was a terrifying experience for the patient who was slipping in and out of consciousness. At that stage, there was no experience base for the future. It was also a frustrating time for doctors who had very few options and a lack of effective drugs.

The days went by in mixed chaos of a pumping iron lung, nursing care of Ilene and hopeless activities. After a few days, my mother and father braved coming to Minneapolis to visit Ilene in the hospital.

It was an overwhelming experience for them and I am sure they concluded that all was lost. Their Finnish-immigrant-community experience was that people went to hospitals to die. They assured me they would do anything I needed to help and returned to their home in Cloquet.

Singing "Beautiful Savior"

In the weeks before Jim was born, we kept contact by just being in the room with Ilene. Ilene appreciated our presence, but drifted off a portion of the time. She expressed joy when I arrived each day. We had a picture of Dan pasted to the front of her lung where she could see the "Beim-Beim" man in his pajamas.

Ilene's father did come to help me in keeping Ilene company, but it was very difficult for him to be in the polio environment. He went back to Ames to his job at the college in the horticulture department and to help take care of the Beim-Beim boy who was now living with his grandparents. Dan received royal treatment from his grandparents and their friends. Harold kept up a very steady line of letters to us and encouraged the family and others to do the same.

During this time I began singing hymns to Ilene. She seemed pleased with my company. I even sang "Beautiful Savior" to her. The conditions were so bad, it probably explained why Ilene could tolerate my singing. I am tone deaf and cannot keep on key. I didn't know all the words, but I knew the meaning. I just ad-libbed the words to the parts that I did not know.

The Birth of James Stanley

Dr. James Bergquist had lost both the mother and the child of the other iron-lung patients. Long days and nights of effort did not succeed. We talked at night of the general problem and of Ilene's condition. She was the least likely to succeed since she could not tolerate the positive-pressure system for breathing that had been employed.

I had noted that the doctors had been viewing her pupils for signals of life. The next morning when I arrived, I noticed a great pile of hospital materials were outside of her room. Dr. Bergquist stated that she appeared to be dying and was "as good as dead." At that moment, Dr. Bergquist initiated a conversation about bypassing saving Ilene's life to go directly to removing our child from her body. He stated it was possible that one life could be saved from the terrible situation. He needed my approval to do so. He wanted approval to take the life of my wife, who was as good as dead, to possibly gain one life.

My decision was immediate. I would not agree to the proposition because we had discussed alternatives and the lack of success to date. I believed people live or die according to God, not by the decisions of men. I also respected Ilene's stated prayer in Note 1 to live to take care of the family:

> *Please pray to God that I have*
> *the faith it takes to make me well and strong.*

Dr. Bergquist understood and did not argue. He stated he would try to develop another plan.

The morning of September 15, 1953, arrived with Dr. Bergquist prepared with another way of delivering the baby. The total procedure was written up and published in a medical journal. Ilene's hospital room was filled with assistants to the delivery. A new manual method of producing breathing was key to the process.

One person operated some type of oxygen bag to introduce pressurized oxygen into Ilene's lungs. I do not know what the other people were doing. Ilene's iron lung was opened with Ilene staying on her iron-lung bed. The process required about a half hour to perform.

The baby was quickly whisked away from the room. I did not have a clue as to the condition of the child. Ilene was reintroduced into the iron lung. I watched the operation from outside the hospital room without knowing the status of the procedure. At the end, I knew Ilene was still alive, in an unknown condition, and that a live child had been delivered. I congratulated a tired-but-happy Dr. James Bergquist on the accomplishment.

After some hours, a nurse came to me and stated I should go to the nursery. When I arrived, a red, wailing baby boy was inside an isolation room. He was kicking and active and very much alive. The nurses were ebullient and joyful. One life had survived!

My immediate reaction was: "Thank God! No matter what happens in my life, I will never give up hope."

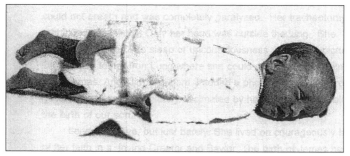

**James, November 15, 1953. The lively baby –
never give up hope.**

CHAPTER 3

Rehabilitation

In 1952, polio was dreaded alongside the fear of the atomic bomb. There was no remedy nor solution to these two problems. Living inside an iron lung was proof that you were an unfortunate victim. Total isolation within the lung was a terrifying, lonely existence. Polio was a dreaded crippler and killer of people. Isolation of its victims was necessary. Minneapolis General Hospital was the Twin Cities facility for the victims. The sixth floor was a polio ward dedicated to the acute cases and the unfortunate who required iron lungs.

Ilene was alive, confined to an iron lung in a small hospital room on the sixth floor. She had been torn from a joyful life in our happy home by the trolley tracks into a fierce, terrifying struggle to survive. A dedicated nurse was constantly attending Ilene 24 hours a day. Ilene could not breathe and was completely paralyzed. Her tracheotomy prohibited her talking. Only her head was outside the lung. She sometimes lapsed into sleep or unconsciousness.

After Jim was born, I added a photo of him to the iron-lung gallery. Ilene was completely decimated by her spinal-bulbar polio and the birth of our son. She lived on courageously because of her faith in a loving Creator and Savior. The birth of James had been the first positive sign for her in two weeks. Yet when I arrived each day, Ilene began to make me realize her love for and pleasure in the visit. She would respond to my presence and the news from the outside world. She especially enjoyed my nightly readings of the Scriptures.

The daily cards and letters from our church and our Augsburg community and our families were most important to Ilene. I needed large boxes to keep them all. They were all read together. Ilene appreciated them all and they provided a happy time every day. The letters contributed to the inner spark and outlook in Ilene that was based upon her faith in God, and our love for each other and for our two boys. But there was no assurance of recovery. It took many days before Ilene was able to leave the lung to sit in a wheelchair. To retain her positive disposition within a hostile environment in which there was only waiting required a great deal of courage. She was not defeated as her faith and her trust in God prevailed. Her prospects improved after our baby was born.

I kept contact by just being in the room with Ilene. The ambiance of noise and tubes, and the constant pumping of the lung were frightening. I tried to bring some normality to the scene. Each day I reviewed the good reports from Ilene's mother about Dan and her father's bright, daily letters. Dan was a big hit in the Ames Arbor Street neighborhood with the good friends of his grandparents.

Our new son appeared to be a very healthy baby who weighed almost five pounds and appeared to have a great amount of energy and vitality. He was named "James" in honor of the physician who attended his birth and who was striving to save his mother's life.

We spent some time in our daily devotions with Bible readings. It was a time without TV or radio. I attempted to sing hymns from memory to Ilene. Since Ilene was musical and had a good ear, it must have been difficult to deal with my off-key attempts.

The hymns I sang served as a means of communication. It probably explained Ilene's acceptance of my singing "Beautiful Savior" to her. Ilene had a keen sense of music but that did not prevent her tolerating a very off- tune singer. Perhaps her tolerance of my singing was based on her sense of humor and that something is better than nothing. Her sense of humor caused her to smile at readings from Mark Twain. We had both studied

German in college and Mark Twain's essay on the German language was funny to both of us.

I had been checking her vital statistics that were posted in a folder attached to her iron lung. After some time, this most discouraging information became a downer to me so I stopped looking at it. We were so far from normal and the information only amplified my concerns related to our status.

I continued to attend Trinity Church near Augsburg. The church was a great support for Ilene and me. One Sunday morning I was approached by an older man who had a dollar bill in his hand when we shook hands. I protested the gift, but he insisted on my accepting it. He had figured out a way of expressing his feelings. His sincerity and his want to show his concern prevailed. I still have the dollar bill in my files. I later was told the man was the father of Ernie Anderson, Augsburg's basketball coach.

Our families became involved in the process of Ilene's condition. Since the Bechtels were in Minneapolis at the time Ilene was first admitted to the hospital, they were intimately knowledgeable of the situation. Ilene's mother, being a nurse, probably had the best grasp of the problem. We agreed that Dan should go home with them and would enjoy being in Ames until a more settled time should come. For me, it was a very painful departure for Dan to go off to Ames. He was dressed in his green-corduroy suit and was happy to be going on a fun car ride. I was sad that he hadn't protested or insisted on staying with me.

Harold went back to work and Blanche was a mother again. The entire neighborhood and social center enjoyed having a happy boy to interact with. Harold started a daily letter to us on Dan's status.

Ilene's Grandmother Bechtel was a unique, intellectual person. She liked to read and could write interesting letters. Several of the letters stated she would write better letters, but they were composed when she was washing dishes and ironing, and somehow lost in subsequent translation.

Ilene' father Harold stayed with me prior to Jim's birth to help in our vigil. It was evident that the situation of watching Ilene was more than he could stand. He returned to Ames to help take care of Daniel. Today, Dan does not remember his time in Ames.

During this time, Bob Kulterman, my best student for several years, taught my introductory physics class.

Helen Bertness volunteered with helping our son Jim transition from the hospital to a home setting. Helen was a member of the Augsburg community. She had experience in raising one of her own premature children. After several weeks of Helen's loving care, Jim was ready for home. Helen's care was part of an overwhelming Augsburg College response to our problem.

The Reverend Martin Olson of Trinity Lutheran Church baptized Jim in our home. Fellow Trinity members, Karl and Addell Dahlen, were his sponsors. They both were faithful godparents and remained interested in James' welfare. Karl was dean of students at Augsburg and Addell was Ilene's friend from the Sunshine Circle at church. My parents, Hannah and Gust, drove down from Cloquet and were present. After the baptism, they took Jim to Cloquet.

There, for the first twelve months of his life, Jim was brought up by loving grandparents. My mother was only in her 40s at that time, and Jim became her second son. It was a very emotional day when she had to part with her Jimmy one year later. My mother had established a comfortable relationship to an assembly-line job and found a new set of friends at the Diamond Match Company. She voluntarily gave up her union rights and her job to take care of Jimmy.

The year that Jim spent in Cloquet was a memorable time in my parents' lives. My mother wrote on May 5, 1953:

> We are all getting along good now.....He has sleep good again two nights already. He sure is getting nicer to take care of....Jimmie sure likes his play pen. He has all his toys there and he sure can move around there. We sure are glad to hear Ilene is improving. It will take time though. You don't have to worry about Jimmie for we sure like him like our own.

Since my father spoke Finnish at home, Jim was a Finnish boy when he was returned to us. My mother took him regularly to be checked by Dr. Butler and Dr. Reino Pumala and his physician wife for medical advice. I managed trips to Cloquet and found James was doing well and my parents were very proud that they could contribute.

It was a time of uncertainty. Ilene was totally dedicated to recovering as much function as possible. I was finishing my fourth year at Augsburg and spent time at the hospital every night.

The battle of the iron lung slowly changed and Ilene began to gain strength. I returned to teaching my classes at Augsburg. A major milestone was Ilene's graduating to a rocking bed. She was first in a wheelchair on October 26, 1952. The doctors had established that Ilene would have a long rehabilitation program ahead with uncertain results. There was doubt about her ability to walk or even whether she could breath on her own. They said it would take months to determine her general status and longer to attain her final capability.

As time went on, it started to become apparent we would need a house where Ilene could best rehabilitate at home. I spent my spare time trying to identify such a place. It was evident we would need some special type of house that could accommodate our needs.

After Ilene was able to sit in a wheelchair, she was transferred to the polio rehabilitation center at Sheltering Arms on the River Road on January 6, 1953. She was able to come home for three days at Christmas. A hospital bed was arranged for this first visit.

The months spent at Sheltering Arms, located on the River Road in Minneapolis, were devoted to hot packs, stretching and exercising the muscle functions that remained. Ilene faced all of this with a fearless courage.

Every night she gave me a bright, joyful greeting and a factual relating of the events of the day. Braces, Kenny Sticks and crutches were fitted and used to rehabilitate functions. The therapists were devoted to their duties but forced to be strict disciplinarians to keep the patients working at their best levels. Ilene worked hard to regain her walking function. Almost all of her normal muscular functions had been affected by the polio.

The patients at Sheltering Arms, through common problems, became a community in themselves. They developed their own vocabulary for the problems. The "#" sign represented their functional ability to operate. I think "0" represented no function. This numerical system graded muscles from being able to overcome gravity to being fully functional, which was a "10."

The patients, however, had their own nomenclature which started with "crudo" (affected) and continued to "el-crudo" (zero).

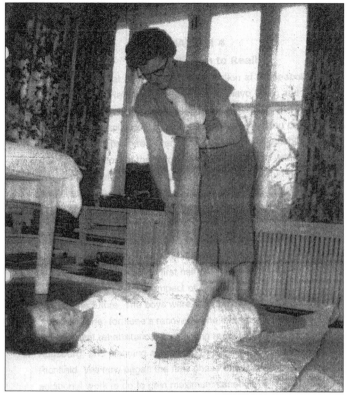

Therapy at Sheltering Arms Hospital.

Such terms were applied to specific functions and to individuals. For example, a person left with little function could be referred to as el-crudo. El Jerome was a slight impairment, hardly significant. Ilene and I retained some of this nomenclature for the rest of our lives. It could be applied to behavior as well as physical attributes.

After intensive therapy, Ilene attempted walking with a special leg brace and crutches in June of that year. It was a very slow walk with an attending therapist at her side. She graduated to the Swedish Rehabilitation Center at the end of July and began discussions with the Mayo Clinic on the type of surgery or treatment that might be helpful. We were making progress, but slowly, and the total extent of recovery was unknown.

An accident happened during Ilene's therapy at Mayo. She was at St. Mary's Hospital undergoing therapy after an operation to improve her walking ability. The children were in Ames for the week. After work, I drove to Mayo for the weekend. I was on a business trip and drove directly to Rochester. I was shocked to find Ilene with a very bruised head and missing front teeth. She had fallen face forward during walking therapy, landing on her face. My initial reaction was one of dismay and, "Who do I sue?" Ilene had stitches in her lips and was black and blue from the fall. However, Ilene's attentions or interests were to alleviate my concerns, my worries. She assured me the therapist was not able to stop her forward fall and that it was not the therapist's fault. Ilene assured me that the dentists were already working on her teeth and that she would be better off than before.

Ilene also said she would like to go to the Mayo Auditorium to hear a Fred Waring concert that night. That was a major thing for Ilene since she was always very conscious of how she appeared, but she wanted to go. We went and enjoyed the concert. This incident was directed toward my welfare and state of mind.

Although I hadn't said a word, she knew what was in my mind and was trying to help me cope with the problem. Her reaction to this problem was a willingness to try everything and live to the fullest extent possible. We did have a good time. Fred Waring had many appearances on TV. In person, it was even better.

We had now spent a year and a half recovering as much as possible from the impact of polio. The formal rehabilitation program was nearing completion. Ilene went through many operations to promote improved movement and some muscle transplants to permit functions or to improve control. These were valuable since she was later able to drive a car with the ability to handle her right foot and to push the brake and throttle.

Ilene had the problem of knowing her two sons were with grandparents. She did not know where she would end up, but it was becoming obvious she would be considerably handicapped. After months of rehabilitation, operations and procedures, the Mayo Clinic doctors had developed a prognosis of Ilene's condition and future. We were informed of two conclusions in a session in Rochester.

The first conclusion was related to walking. They felt Ilene's muscle capability and control was too limited to be able to walk with any practical value. They felt she would never be able to lift her foot over any obstacle, even small doorsteps. Ilene had conscientiously practiced at home as well at hospitals to gain a walking capability. The effort was however very difficult and tedious. Further, the doctors felt it would be a waste of her energy that could better be used in taking care of our two boys. The doctors felt the quality of Ilene's life would be better when confined to her wheelchair.

The second conclusion related to Ilene's breathing deficiencies. The doctors told us that Ilene was primarily breathing via her diaphragm. She had no breathing via her chest muscles. The consequence of this was that we should not plan on having more children. A baby in her abdomen would restrict her diaphragm breathing, risking the viability of the child and her own survival. This conclusion was a difficult one for us, as we had always wanted at least four children.

CHAPTER 4

Reconciliation to Reality

After the year and a half of rehabilitation at Minneapolis General, Sheltering Arms Rehabilitation Center and the Swedish Hospital, we began the construction of the pattern for our life. We were zero prepared to evaluate our situation and bring our two sons back home. In all of this, Ilene resolutely did her very best to recover and always retained a positive outlook. She was determined to become a mother to our two boys, an answer to her prayer in her "Note One" to me.

Ilene was a victim of bulbar-spinal polio, which meant her breathing capability and physical handicaps were severe and well established. We were told that most of the recovery would take place within a year. It was possible to provide some aid and techniques to assist in muscle rehabilitation and specific aids to some movements. Nothing could be done with respect to breathing.

It is difficult to see the reality that faced Ilene. She was a realist who reacted to her world. The long rehabilitation process had been all encompassing. Whereas I had a new job at Honeywell that was interesting, Ilene could not estimate what her ability to interact with the outside world would be. How Ilene would be able to be a mother to her boys and maintain the home were a total unknown. We started with a full-time aide, Eunice Johnson. She was the neighbor who was related to the Augsburg family and who did not have children at that time. After a six-month period, we hired a full-time housekeeper for one day a week.

Our little house by the trolley tracks was a very small one on a half lot. It had major steps at the entrance. Through friends at Trinity Church, we found a builder-architect in a major housing development. He redesigned one of his track houses to meet our needs. The Mattson Builders were completing the work on our new house at 7501-11th Avenue in Richfield. The architect's son spent considerable effort to include the latest means of making a handicapped-accessible house for a wheelchair occupant. This included having sliding doors for interior rooms to permit maximum-width entries for all rooms. The natural cork floors were chosen to also aid walking practice. Working areas in the kitchen were 30 inches high.

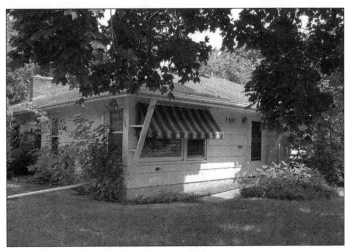

Our home in Richfield.

A built-in stove was kept to a depth of single burner to help reach cooking utensils. A washer and dryer were added to the kitchen to minimize travel for washing. This was accomplished by eliminating one of the standard bedrooms. Additional closets and storage facilities were added. The house was landscaped to eliminate steps for entry while maintaining a normal appearance. Exterior windows were enlarged and lowered to permit Ilene to observe the boys in the yard.

Ilene had to familiarize herself with all the needed work in a totally new environment. She also had to develop a plan or method to accomplish the needed tasks.

The realities of having the means to build a new special house and to support an unknown future became apparent. Without any effort on our part we were presented with a means to work the problem. In retrospect, it seemed that God was providing an answer.

Elmer Frykman of Honeywell heard of my problems. He talked to me and suggested that I consider taking a job in his Field Service School until I had a better handle on my true needs. Elmer was a graduate of Augsburg who heard of our problems via his college friends. I accepted the offer from a very kind and friendly man who later became my friend. We understood the possibility that I would return to college teaching if it were possible. I would start at Honeywell when the school year was over in June.

We entered a new phase of life in the fall of 1953. We had spent the remainder of 1952 and the first half of 1953 in intensive rehabilitation, recovering from the initial impact of polio and determining what could be done in the future. The children were with their grandparents to create a time to provide a maximum condition for Ilene. In addition to rehabilitation for Ilene, I was occupied with completing my teaching assignments at Augsburg and planning and starting the building of our new home in Richfield. Ilene still had additional work to do to gain maximum capability and we had to prepare the house for occupancy.

Our old house in Minneapolis was sold and our furniture stored at my cousin Harold's garage in Bloomington. I stayed at Harold's for a short time in transition to the new home. But then a new life started for us as we assimilated to our realities.

Our Plymouth had a poor heater so in preparation for cold weather travel, I traded it in for a pea-green 1950 Nash with a great heater and a very bulbous shape. We began to take short weekend trips to see the boys. It was called a "Bloomer Nash" by Grandpa Harold which was pronounced "Blooming Nash" by our boys.

Working at Honeywell was the source of interesting topics. The people I interacted with were a surprise. Arne Matthies had been a physics teacher at Luther College in Iowa and came to Honeywell to help support his large family. John Maynard was a devout Baptist with a bright outlook on life.

Elmer Frykman had a great deal of experience in Honeywell field service as well as being a former "Augie." He taught me how to play chess and needled me after he had beaten me and I stated "I had the better position." It turned out my experiences at Honeywell would be positive and we met many friends who would become our mutual friends.

CHAPTER 5

Transition to Stability

At the onset of her illness, Ilene had written:

I long with all my being to be back
with you and take care of you.

Please pray to God that I have
the faith it takes to make me well
and strong.

Ilene was discharged from the Sheltering Arms rehabilitation hospital in September 1953 but continued to work with doctors to improve her capabilities. Neurotripsies were performed to increase the functions in functioning muscle groups. We went to the Mayo Clinic for operations to improve her ability to control her feet that would enable her to drive a car.

In the fall of 1954, after 18 months of struggle in institutions, we wondered whether Ilene could fit into a totally new environment with two young boys, a new house, new friends and a need to find her role? Could she do so despite her significant physical handicaps and mental trauma? It would require emotional stability and courage. It was now Ilene's time of reality for dealing with our problems.

Our builder-architect, Mattson, drew up plans for a significant modification to his track houses. We seldom discussed the limitations and problems with our two sons, preferring to do what we could to live our lives fully within our restrictions. This was probably a questionable position as it also carried into their behavior of not sharing some of their problems with us.

The windows designed by Mattson enabled Ilene to see out and monitor the boys and their friends playing. The boys were accustomed to having a loving mother in a wheelchair, and seldom gave us a problem. They accepted our situation as a normal one. The house was slightly larger than the track houses and eliminated one bedroom. New features that accommodated Ilene's wheelchair introduced three-foot-wide sliding doors, lower enlarged windows for visibility and new kitchen facilities including 30-inch-high counter heights. The architect's plan provided an open house that could be used for Ilene's walking exercise. She could use a circular circuit in the house for walking with crutches. The house had an open, spacious feeling. Although it was a special-built house, the builder sold it to us at a modest additional cost to the houses he was building. I am sure the cost of the house was more than our purchase price.

As soon as we were in the new house, Ilene began her walking exercises around the obstruction-free track that we had established. Ilene accommodated to the new electric stoves and washer-dryer in the kitchen. The everyday living requirements were very tiring to Ilene.

Ilene was not able to visit neighbors' houses nor establish many neighbor-to-neighbor social contacts. Conversely, the neighboring wives did not visit with Ilene because they never met her in yard activities and neighbor-to-neighbor talk. Since we had a daytime housekeeper for our home for several months, it was not necessary to for neighbors offer aid either.

Although Ilene did not often relate to the women in the neighborhood, she stuck up for her boys when they were scolded by a neighbor mother or when they were accused of misbehavior. She also was an apt referee for any disagreements that transpired between her two boys.

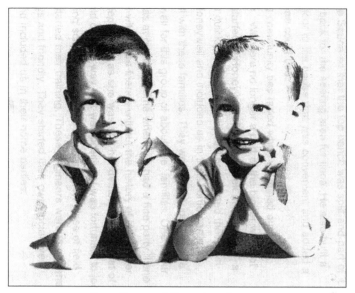

Sons Dan and Jim return home.

We modified the original house by adding a garage and finished the basement to build bedrooms for our sons. We quickly added a double garage to facilitate transfer from car to wheelchair and provide all-weather entry to the house.

The garage was built to accommodate a sauna that my father personally designed with a great deal of care. It included benches that allowed Ilene to sit comfortably in a position the shower could reach. He wrote me a note, the only note he ever wrote me, with detailed instructions on how to heat up the sauna. He also included a spare "quias" (heating stove) to ensure long-time operation.

Our garage was planned to have only a one-car capability since I felt a Finnish sauna would be a much-welcomed addition. As soon as the garage was in place, my father took vacation time to build the sauna. It was earlier than I planned since funds were short, but my father wanted to make his contribution.

My father had the sauna all planned and brought the sauna stove with him from Cloquet. He ordered the lumber from the local lumber company. It was first class and expensive. This was a short-term problem we lived with. He planned the sauna so that Ilene could attend in comfort. He also built ramping from the car door to the house that was convenient and added a low handrail that Ilene could use.

Ilene found the house very compatible to her needs and it enabled us to bring our children home to an adequate, even commodious place. The house had been a major reason for my move to work at Honeywell and it proved to be a good answer to some problems.

Our Boys Return Home

The boys' grandparents brought the children back home in two steps. Dan arrived first from Ames. He seemed to fit in right away and was very much at home. Ilene's parents had a social life in which Dan was included. He was the "King of the Hill" to a lot of people, including his great-grandparents Herb and Estelle who wrote:

> *"Danny is a darling. He does such funny things*
> *for such a little guy. If I were 40 years younger,*
> *I don't think Ilene would have Danny...."*

My parents brought Jim home a week or so later. Jim had been brought up in a very isolated Finnish "atmosphere" in Cloquet. My parents continued to speak Finnish at home as my father never became fluent in English. My mother brought Jim up from infancy and took on the role of his mother. So the transition for Jim was larger. Some of his initial vocabulary was Finnish. Since Finnish had been my own original language, I was able to ease his transition.

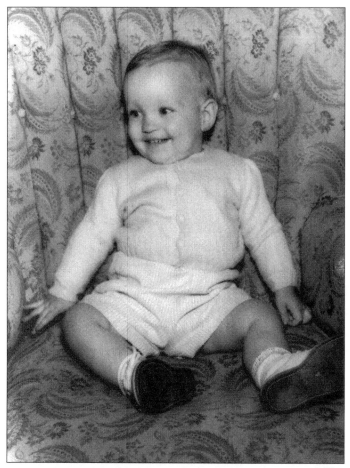

Son Jim when he left Cloquet.

The two brothers also had the issue of getting to know each other and learning how to play together. Fortunately, our new neighborhood was full of friendly children their age so it did not require much at that time. The boys were very attentive to Ilene's restrictions and this provided a means for their outdoor activity. So we had a transition to an interesting new world in which Ilene could participate and enjoy life. The key elements were her transparent friendliness (the Essential Ilene) and her effort to contribute within her capability.

Our first household helper was Eunice Johnson, wife of an accountant at Augsburg. Eunice worked for a period as a full-time day assistant. Our boys were one- and two-year olds when they returned home from their loving grandparents. They both do not claim to remember their experience with their grandparents. They only knew a mother who was in a wheelchair who had to establish relationships. Ilene had a faith and trust in a loving God who knew her and her problems. Her only method of rebuilding relationships had to be based upon love and her own radiance of being. The boys seemed to accept their relations to their mother and were mostly obedient to her instructions.

The boys stayed off the streets and played within her sight. The windows in our house were oversized with a low bottom sill so Ilene could observe the boys' outside activities. Indeed, she seemed to know everything that went on up and down 11th Avenue. Dick Pearson, whom Ilene fondly called "Pearie," commented that nothing went on that she didn't see from her "perch" in the window.

When we first moved in, the Badens lived next door with two little girls with whom our boys had great fun. The Laces lived across the street with Bob, Joey, John and later Margit. Pearie lived a few houses down the street and became a most important friend in Jim's life. Our back yard was a playground for baseball, football and basketball. I played with the boys while Ilene confined her games to indoor ones.

Ilene devised a way of doing things at home within her capability. She could transport the boys to little league baseball with help with the wheelchair. The boys learned to help with transporting Mother. Each would take hold of a side of the wheelchair and provide a major pull that enabled us to easily take major hills and rough terrain in good style. We were able to handily attend events that had long and inclined ramps. This teamwork was also an extraordinary mark on Ilene's taking the role of the leader of the home. I have asked my sons now, later in life, if they were limited by their mother's handicaps. Without hesitation, the answer was no. Ilene's friends were also able to relate to a caring person, not to her handicaps.

Ilene was able to fit into a new environment with two winsome sons and a new house. This she was able to do without lamenting what she could not do or regretting her deficiencies. This ability to live courageously within her capabilities would be established. Her faith in God's providence grew.

Ilene became the mother of the house in every sense. She planned the meals and organized the family schedules for our home. Church was an integral part of these plans. The boys began to branch out to lives of their own with respect to friends and organized activities. My work schedules at Honeywell, which was more than 10 miles away, required that I leave in the morning and return home for a happy family supper. Ilene now managed a housekeeper, Mrs. Davidson, who could fill in for the work Ilene could not do herself. Ilene directed her efforts to what she could do and thereby allowed her access and achievement. She never felt it necessary to bewail what she could not do, but she had to deal realistically with problems associated with that.

Church

In 1954 we began looking for a new church. Old Trinity Lutheran Church by Augsburg had a construction in which entry to the building was via many exterior steps and the interior had many restrictions incompatible to wheelchairs. The choir loft was out of the question for a wheelchair, making it impossible for Ilene to participate in something very important to her.

Our ties to Trinity were still very real to us. Karl and Addell Dahlen were special friends. The Sunshine Circle at Trinity church selected material, fabricated and installed our living room drapes. They were a handsome set of curtains that matched the coloring of the room. They were vertically striped dark brown and tan that were from the top of the windows to just below the windowsills. They were complementary to the two natural oak walls, which our builder had added to a living room to make it warm and friendly.

One of our first actions was to locate a church that had accessible facilities. My cousin Harold and his wife Mary had just joined a Lutheran Mission Church in Bloomington – Grace Lutheran. It was established and funded as a starter building on 85th Street and Cedar Avenue. The building was without stairs or a basement and was a new congregation led by Reverend James Christensen, a recent seminary graduate. In a sense, all of us were starting anew. We found a very hospitable community, many of whom were new to church life and especially friendly to us. It provided a forward-looking new environment for our family. Except for Harold and Mary, our past history was not known.

Ilene's normal brightness, our two young sons and a young Honeywell engineer were part of the forward atmosphere of Grace. Ilene seemed to radiate friendliness and a happy disposition. The church was a few minutes from our house and was completely wheelchair compatible. This brought in another circle of friends, quite different from our Augsburg or college crowd. We were welcomed and fit in well with a more diverse set of people. We were part of the original founders of the church. All of us had a new experience with which to acclimate. Ilene was able to teach Sunday school, sing in the choir and participate in the church community. She was recruited to play piano for some Sunday school functions and the social life of the church. We bought a spinet piano so Ilene could practice at home.

We made friends with several of the families in the congregation including strong ties with the Reuben Leruds. Dorlie Lerud was the director of the choir; Reuben was involved in the church headquarters and had a background in church affairs. Pastor Jim loved golf, so I joined a regular Saturday morning round at the Fort Snelling golf course. Grace Lutheran was an ideal church for our family as we transitioned out of the Augsburg community, which still provided us with friends and events to follow.

Our young pastor, James Christensen, had ideas related to how a new church should be organized and operated. A major element was in having one fund-raising activity during the year and avoiding all other fund raising activities. We participated in the new church development and it provided a creative element to our lives at the time. For a number of years, many of us continued the friendships to New Years' parties and the interchange of information about our children. Our new world was interesting and occupied our happy family.

Work Life

The Augsburg community ties faded when we joined our local church and I took my new job at Honeywell. We were no longer an active part of the bigger world of academia. Dr. Otto Schmitt of the biophysics department talked to me about continuing toward a biophysics doctorate at of the U of M. Although we were now operating within our income, it did not appear possible to return to Augsburg in any near future.

Since I started at Honeywell after test week at Augsburg, a new dimension was added to our lives. I was fortunate to join the training school at the same time as a new class of field service engineers started their training. These engineers were young men who were gregarious and friendly. They started their own social lives within Honeywell and included us in their home parties. Ilene fit in well with these families.

One of our social gatherings was at our new home where we

had a fine party. Ilene was able to interact with these friends without the history of her former condition. They accepted her as she was and her demeanor was that of doing what she could do, in a way that was positive. We also started friendships with members of the Honeywell Training School. So our lives rapidly took on a new dimension, which permitted us to have new friends and interests.

These new friends did not have past history or memories of Ilene. People who knew a young, vivacious girl with physical capabilities tended to have a feeling of what was now lost or would be lost in our lives. These people saw Ilene as she was – a friendly, joyful lady in a wheelchair.

Her identity was fresh to these people and gave Ilene the opportunity to begin living a new life within her capabilities. She was the neat wife of another new member of the Honeywell engineers. The class knew her as the person she was – not the person she wasn't.

Honeywell of 1953 was a young, expanding company with many growth opportunities for young engineers and returning servicemen. The five young, new trainees were in a similar boat. We all needed friends and social activities in our new work environment. Only Ken Barlow was single in this group. At the time, he drove a Cadillac Coupe that was made useful for his bachelor life.

Being an instructor, the Field Service School was my first assignment at Honeywell. It was a good assignment since it dealt within all the systems that were in the operational fields. They ranged from the first C1 autopilot used in WWII bombers to the latest fuel-gage systems. The courses were well designed and emphasized knowing enough of the engineering behind the design of the equipment for auto pilots, fuel gauges, etc., that helped understand the systems.

Vacations

My Honeywell job provided the means to arrange for vacations interesting to everyone in our family. The boys became efficient at helping with the wheelchair and in making plans for our trips. The increased awareness of the needs for handicapped facilities began to impact hotel/motel accommodations and public buildings.

Before bicycles were available to the boys, Ilene had been able to drive a car with some special features. Her right side was able to operate thanks to several operations on her feet and arms. The boys and Ilene developed schemes to help her access the car and handle the folding wheelchair.

By choosing wide-door coupes equipped with power assists and leather seats, Ilene could work into the driver's seat. The boys would fold the chair and introduce it into the car. Vacation trips during the summer were especially fun and joyful.

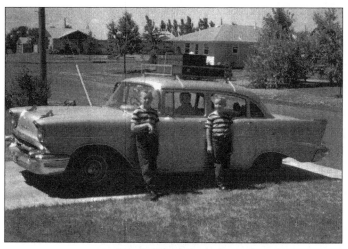

Start of vacation trip.

Key to the success of our vacations was planning them within our capability as a family and having the right facilities available. The boys were interested in motels having swimming pools and Mom and Dad sought large bathrooms. The 1960–1965 vacations were planned to include our total two-week vacation allotment. It took some time to acclimatize to our family apart from work and routine activities. Two weeks of time facilitated the establishment of the family together. The longer period was available before the boys' independent activities prohibited them from joining Ilene and me.

We purchased a 1961 Chevy station wagon and installed a large luggage rack on top. The result was a large, level floor in the wagon for the boys to play and to have naps. We were a most compatible traveling group. Ilene was very happy to travel and enjoy life. We took enough pictures of our trips that one gets the sense of having family fun together. The boys were very compatible and could entertain each other with various activities and "adventures."

A Western Trip to South Dakota with Morris and Ivey

Our first major family vacation trip was to Morris and Ivey's home in the Black Hills of South Dakota. Morris was Ilene's father's closest cousin. Harold and Morris had enjoyed a good, long-time relationship. Morris suggested we spend time with them just outside Rapid City. He was a horticulturist in the area who had a large, Western-style home in a scenic setting. Morris and his wife Ivey made a special effort to accommodate our family and make our visit memorable.

The boys rode ponies and stage coaches. We searched for the lost gold mine Morris "knew." After a rough drive in the hills, over rivers and non-highway paths, we accidentally found the mine in the hills although the gold was not available to us. We all went to a melodrama. We visited twice, the second time with cousin Gary, and included the famous statues of the presidents.

The Black Hills trips established that we could manage and have a great deal of fun in so doing, due in part to Ilene's courageous "can do" spirit. The two boys were beginning to provide help that enabled us to handle outdoor activities.

A Trip to the Civil War Battlefields

The Civil War Centennial Celebration provided the basis for our 1961 vacation. We started the trip with visits to the Purcells in Madison and the Fishers in Chicago. Ilene was enabled to participate in the activities we chose to see, so it began to be a most pleasant family-building trip. Aunt Bess, Ilene's favorite aunt, helped make the visits most pleasant.

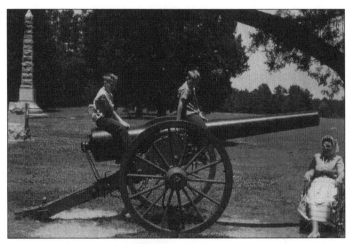

The cannoneers.

One tradition on the vacations was the need to take a "cannon" picture with every cannon in the landscapes. The Civil War gave us ample opportunity to have the boys assume various poses with the many cannons of the battlefields. One special occasion was having Mother in the picture guiding the artillery men.

We visited most of the major battlefields and their diorama explanations. With some care, we were able to travel comfortably. We visited battlefields such as Antietam and Gettysburg, and the museums of Washington, D.C., and Richmond, Virginia.

Our visit to the U.S. Capital building was highlighted by a chance meeting with Minnesota Senator Hubert Humphrey. While waiting for me to park the car, a capital attendant asked Ilene where we were from. Upon finding out we were from Minnesota, he asked her to wait for a short time because he knew Senator Humphrey would be arriving and would want to see us. We had a picture taken of the senator and our family, a major highlight.

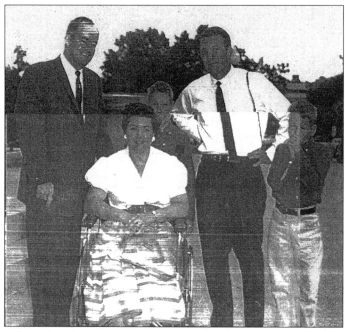

We visit with Minnesota Senator Hubert H. Humphrey while vacationing in Washington, D.C.

Disneyland, Seattle and a Pullman Ride on the Empire Builder

One of Ilene's achievements was to enable me to make necessary business trips for Honeywell. With the help of the two boys, she was capable of short periods of total independence. This was especially important once I assumed technical management on some NASA Space Shuttle programs. With the help of the boys and a well-planned agenda she worked out, Ilene took pride in being a help to me in these matters. I arranged the trips to facilitate our needs. From the standpoint of the boys, I am sure they viewed this as normal procedure. Later they began to see the enormous courage and self confidence necessary for their mother to enable me to do my job. She never claimed she was doing something unusual, although she was.

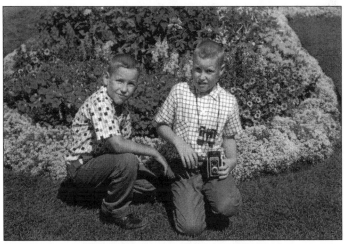

Posing by a pretty flower garden.

Our California trip was our grand tour trip. I had to attend an Apollo design review at North American Aviation in Downey, California. We planned a vacation "grand tour" around the meeting. We flew first class on a DC-7 and stayed at the Tahitian Village Motel in Downey. It was the first airline trip for the boys. The multi-day review required that Ilene and the boys fend for themselves for a couple of days. A great swimming pool gave the boys something pleasant to do. We went one night to the Angels baseball game with our Minnesota Twins. North American provided us with some tickets to Disneyland. We enjoyed spending the tickets although we had trouble using them all up.

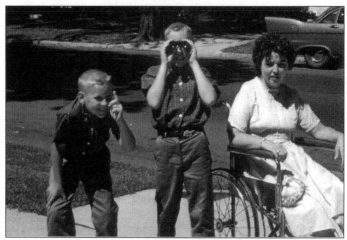

Looking for something while on vacation.

We rented a station wagon very similar to our own and began the scenic trip to Seattle, stopping along the way to stay at swimming-pool equipped motels. Seattle had just finished with the World's Fair so there were plenty of sites to visit.

We took the famous Empire Builder train back home to Minneapolis. This was the Great Northern Railway's flagship train originated by the empire builder himself, James J. Hill. This train had been updated in 1962. We rented a double-bedroom, one-compartment sleeper room so we could enjoy to scenic trip.

I had to carry Ilene onto the train, but it was a memorable occasion. We took our meals in our compartment. Ilene was able to maintain her bright and joyful outlook for the total trip. It was quite a trip that required a lot of patience on her part.

The conclusion of these trips was also the completion of grade school for the boys. This period also was the most enjoyable time as a family. We had formed a Christian family in which Ilene was an essential part. She managed the home in which each family member had a happy part.

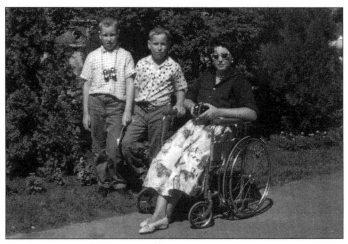

Team "Ready to roll."

Chapter 6

Full Family Life

The boys completed elementary school and began to have independent activities. It became more difficult to arrange long periods of time for vacations. In 1963, we transferred to Woodlake Lutheran Church in Richfield so as to enable the boys to attend church with school friends. Woodlake was very wheelchair compatible. The Christian membership and pastoral staff were friendly and understanding. Ilene and I found many activities and people to be compatible with. In short, we were able to live a full life despite Ilene's physical handicaps. This took place rather rapidly due to a large extent to Ilene's ability to project her essential nature and faith in a friendly manner. Friends soon forgot that Ilene was handicapped, thinking of her as a total person. This situation prevailed from our boys' grade school years through high school. Countless prayers had been answered as she had asked for at the onset of polio.

> *I long with all my being to be back*
> *with you and take care of you.*

Ilene was a person who had the understanding that God had answered the prayers of many. She was handicapped but was able to take care of the tasks she was given. She was the Essential Ilene, a radiant person.

Ilene was again in the church choir, singing in the alto section. She also developed a unique, close relationship to Pearl Sorenson. Pearl began to visit Ilene weekly or when I was on a trip.

Later, we had planned to move to a more spacious home, again designed by Mattson, but our two boys preferred to stay at the current location so as to retain their friends and school arrangements. We have lived in the same house together for over 55 years.

Ilene and I began attending the new Guthrie Theater in 1964. We purchased season tickets for years and attended most all of the plays from the opening play "Hamlet" with George Grizzard to the closing play at the old Guthrie, which also was "Hamlet." We both enjoyed attending the plays and usually ate supper at the theater before the play. For a number of years, we had a group of Honeywell friends attend on the same night and then gathered at the Lincoln Del on Lake Street to discuss the play. Ilene was always an interesting play partner as she viewed plays from a different perspective.

Later we extended our play going to the Penumbra Theater in St. Paul, where we again had season tickets. We also had fun going to the Old Log Theater comedies and the Minnesota Centennial Showboat melodramas. These and other theater experiences were especially important to us as we could enjoy them fully despite the wheelchair restrictions.

Ilene continued the major responsibility for the running and the conduct of agendas within our home. Obviously she was not able to do certain things, but the house plan was well thought out by the builder and permitted a maximum of participation. The laundry facility in the kitchen helped her wash and dry clothes efficiently. She planned meals according to the needs of our various schedules. Her cooking facilities were accessible to her and permitted her to cook meals. At a later time she was able to cook multiple meals due to the participation of the boys in various activities and my own work uncertainties.

Ilene always cooked a hot breakfast for her family. She sent her family off into the world warm and with satisfied appetites. Jim has continued this tradition from her motherly model even to this present day. He usually provides a warm morning breakfast for his wife and children, and sometimes even to his grandchildren when they are in his home.

One of Ilene's independent activities was singing in choirs. She was involved in church choirs all the years of our marriage. She had a good alto voice and appreciated most music. An exception was some of Sibelius' symphonies, which she found depressing. One of her most independent activities for Ilene was singing in the Richfield Mother Singers. Not only did she enjoy the singing but also the company of a diverse group of women. She made friends that continued after she was unable to participate.

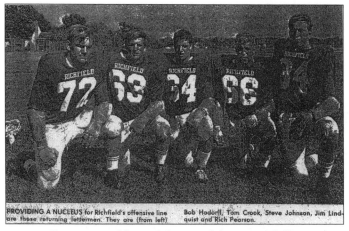

PROVIDING A NUCLEUS for Richfield's offensive line are those returning lettermen. They are (from left) Bob Hodorff, Tom Crook, Steve Johnson, Jim Lindquist and Rich Pearson.

Jim – second from right, number 66 – with his
Richfield High School football buddies.

Son James became very involved in high school football. He was not big, but was very strong and fast. Ilene attended most of his games at Richfield High School and later at Augsburg College. It was vexing to be forced to sit at ground level for most of the high school games and all Augsburg games at the old Parade Stadium in Minneapolis. It was also tough to have such poor seats on the sidelines when people would stand up and obstruct her view during the most exciting times. Her circulation, which had never been great, became even poorer due to her inability to move her legs.

Ilene's parents attended a ceremony for the "All Lake Conference" football team. Ilene and I attended an awards dinner at the Minneapolis Club in downtown Minneapolis. Jim was selected for the team. At that time, the Lake Conference was the most prestigious football conference in the state.

Another family highlight was the selection of Jim to be the 1970 "Richfield High School Scholar-Athlete of the Year." This was most meaningful to our family. Jim won the award in a large high school with a lot of competition from athletes of various sports. Although Ilene was most joyous and proud of Jim's accomplishments, she provided a realistic world that required Jim to have a meaningful perspective.

Ilene and I treasured Dan's music accomplishments. We attended as many of Dan's public appearances as possible and we enjoyed them greatly. Dan wrote a number of songs including the "Banana Song." Later, while Ilene was hospitalized for the last time, Jim brought in the "Banana Song" for her to listen to. Ilene and Jim happily reminisced about the band and the past experiences with the song.

As I continued at Honeywell, we developed lasting friendships with many families. Ilene was highly admired and was a joyful participant in social life. These friendships have continued to this day. This is especially true of the circle of friends surrounding the Apollo Project at Honeywell. Joanne and Peter Lundquist were special friends. He is an excellent artist who has provided us with artwork in our home. One of his paintings is that of an early wade by Ilene and me in a creek in Ledges State park in Boone, Iowa. Pete painted it from a photograph taken on an early college date.

Another good friend has been Linc Hudson whom we also met when I worked on the Apollo Project. Linc and Ilene became "cousins" via some connection to General Winfield Scott of the Civil War.

Linc and Ilene shared an interest in baseball in which Ilene was the possessor of mystic knowledge of the Minnesota Twins. Ilene's baseball background extended back to Pawnee, Nebraska, where the family followed the town baseball team. Her grandfather Herb was an outstanding first baseman who was forever hurt by not being able to join the Chicago White Sox for a playing opportunity.

Ilene was interested in baseball before we met. Her family attended local Ames city team games in which the catcher was a family friend. Harley Wilhem was also a professor and well-known atomic scientist who has a building named after him at Iowa State University. His daughter Lorna was a classmate of Ilene's who still plays in alumni bands.

When we first moved to Minneapolis, we followed and attended some Minneapolis Miller's games. The Millers were an affiliate of the New York Giants. We watched an exciting outfielder named Willie Mays climb walls to catch fly balls until he was recalled to lead the Giants to pennants.

Ilene was a real fan who maintained her interest in the Minnesota Twins in good times and bad. It was an interest we shared with Linc Hudson. We both bought tickets to the 1964 World Series with the understanding that probably only one of us would get tickets. We used our two tickets to have our boys attend one game and Ilene and I attended the other. Jim Katt out dueled Sandy Koufax in the game we saw, a real thrill for baseball fans such as Ilene and me. This interest continued and gave us fertile ground for talking about important things such as winning two World Series.

Ilene attended many high school functions. She was at most of
son Jim's games despite the cold weather, rain and terrible viewing
of games from the sidelines. She endured the cold winds and elements quietly despite poor circulation in her affected extremities.
She worked with me to devise methods to stay warm. Cold and
inclement weather or poorly accessible stands rarely kept her
away from Jim's games. When something interesting happened,
it was most likely obscured to Ilene by sideline people who stood
up to see what was happening.

Jim's wrestling career was also on our attendance lists. Jim
was not so enthused about this very difficult and sometimes
offensive sport. He was a captain of the championship team in
his senior year.

After his high school graduation, Jim chose to attend Augsburg
College so he could continue to play football with his friends. By
his senior year, Jim decided he had had enough of football. His
college friends, especially neighbor Dick Pearson, visited Ilene to
help convince Jim to play. Ilene would not promote him playing,
saying that football was just a game. Jim did play his final year,
which turned out to be one of Augsburg's best seasons.

Son Dan grew into a kind, loving person who could make
friends. He sprained his knee in 8th-grade football which stopped
his pursuit of sports. He was bright and intelligent had a good
sense of humor.

Dan was with the high school band and was much involved in
music groups. He began to take lessons on trombone in conjunc-
tion with his high school band. His teacher recommended him to
the leader of the Lake Calhoun VFW performing marching band,
a top band in the area. It was active in many summer festivals,
including the Aquatennial parades.

Dan enjoyed the music and was a young member of one of the
outstanding marching bands that won many awards. Ilene and

I enjoyed attending many of their events including out-of-town parades.

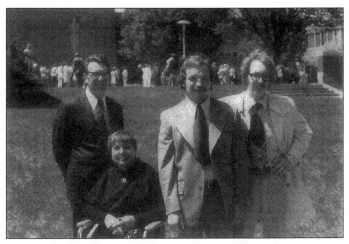

Jim's graduation from Augsburg College – 1974.

Dan took a fancy to playing the guitar and performed in many bands. One of the first was a local neighborhood garage band of young scholars. Dan was recruited at church for various functions that led to him being invited to join John Ylvisaker's band that traveled to churches within the metro area. Ylvisaker was also a composer whose work is included in the Evangelical Lutheran Worship hymnal used in our church. He recently received an honorary doctorate from Wartburg College.

Dan made an out-state trip that interfered with his senior prom. His girlfriend of the moment accompanied the band. Ilene and I attended one of the concerts at a Catholic church in Stillwater. This was the home church of my long-time Honeywell friend Joe Miller.

Dan later became a member of the Rudy Lopez Rock Band. The band practiced in our basement in its organizing stages with the blessing of Ilene. She enjoyed the "rock- and-roll" music that they played. Ilene strongly supported the band. The band called her "Peach." Peach seemed to be a very appropriate name for the chief band supporter. She was first named Peach, inspired by the rock duo "Peaches and Herb," by Dick Pearson, a friend of our son Jim.

Ilene was able to enjoy the passage of the 1970s as much as any other mother. The growing-up years through high school were especially joyous for our family. Ilene enabled her family the same opportunities as any one could want.

Each of the boys was confirmed and brought up the in a warm Christian home. Ilene was happy with her ability to permit her boys a measure of independence.

I was given the opportunity to work in a progressive-but-time-demanding work environment at Honeywell. This included working more than five years on the exciting Apollo Moon Program. I was invited to make presentations about this in Europe and Japan.

Center to all of our activities, Ilene maintained a daily prayer life, Bible study and time given to her Lord Jesus Christ. This was an unobtrusive life that did not demand compliance or special attention. Her greetings and first touch of the day were radiant and loving. Her love and joy were transparent to many.

The years through the 1980s were very special to our family. The boys graduated from high school in 1968 and 1969 and began their independent living. Jim married Ruth in 1976 after graduating from Augsburg College. He found employment at a hospital as an accountant while Ruth finished her degree in nursing at the University of Minnesota.

Dan married Krista in 1977. It was a joyous event for our family. This photo of Ilene at the groom's dinner captures the joy very well. Unfortunately, Dan's marriage ended in divorce and he moved to San Francisco to start a new life. He was able to find work as an electronic technician in the then-flourishing hi-fi world. As this activity became more restrictive, he started taking courses in local colleges which eventually led to a masters degree in math from the University of California in Berkley. He taught high school mathematics for a time. When Dan went to California, he continued to play with Dave Costa, a professional musician in San Francisco.

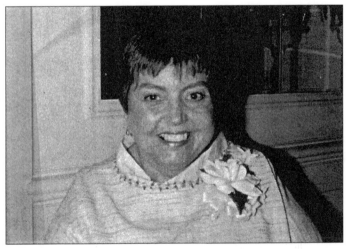

Joyful Ilene at Dan's wedding dinner.

We considered ourselves very fortunate to have been enabled to bring up our boys and to have given them a start despite the trauma of the 1950s. Ilene's composure and spirit had prevailed. She was a rock and certainly had been given the strength she had prayed for.

Chapter 7

Family Building – Living in a Real World

By the time the boys completed grade school, we had established our "normal" family operating procedures. Ilene's physical limitations were established and could be handled. My Honeywell job was challenging and interesting and provided the means needed for raising our family. The boys progressed through grade school with a loving mother. The wheelchair was a part of normal family life.

As we moved into the 1980s, the boys became more independent and involved in defining their own lives. Our family ties remained strong. We attended church regularly to worship God. Christ was the basis for our faith. Ilene was joyfully central to this and her love was given without rancor or scolding. As a close family, we enjoyed Sundays that frequently included being together with friends.

Ilene's role and contribution to this period is a victorious celebration of human achievement. Her life was based on her belief in God and the love of her Savior Jesus Christ. She daily studied the Bible and prayed in her private devotions. Physically, she had severe overall weakness. She had some capability on her right side but her left side was severely weakened and she had limited breathing capability. She was, however, determined to contribute to her family and to do whatever she could do with joy. She did this without drawing notice to her problems or weaknesses. Her limitations were handled as a matter of normal life. As a consequence, our family enjoyed love and life.

The contributions of Ilene were a normal part of a family that experienced many activities. At the same time her participation and contributions required a great number of personal achievements that were taken for granted as normal. Some of her major personal achievements are noted below.

Family Worship and Church

Ilene was central to the establishment of a Christian home that had discipline and substance. Schedules were met as she planned. This required Ilene to be far ahead in her own preparations. There was never any doubt as to our intent or participation nor was there forcing or coercion.

Regular attendance at Woodlake Lutheran Church provided a major joy and happiness to our lives. Our Christian friendships and fellowship were basic to our living. Sunday worship was usually followed by our lunches at The Good Earth or other favorite eating places. Many of our Woodlake friends came with us. The manager of the restaurant, "Newmie" (Kathy Neuman), was a member of our son's church in Bloomington. As regular customers, we became friends of the staff and other regulars.

A frequent 30-mile trip to the Lavender Inn in Faribault was a happy event. Easter and Christmas celebrations in our homes were greatly looked forward to and enjoyed. Ilene's love and concern were always evident. Easter-egg contests with the children were especially precious to Grandma Peach. She was the person around which the grand contests were enjoyed.

Another example of the love shared between Ilene and her children, grandchildren and great-grandchildren was during the annual Easter-egg contests. The competition in the egg-cracking contest was exciting. The eggs of the contestants met in a joyful and lively uproar of fun and intent to crack the egg held by the other. On these occasions, Peach held her own. Whether or not she won or they "defeated" her, all who were present deeply sensed her love and interest in them.

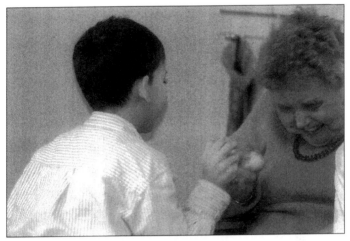

Easter egg contest.

Home Management

Ilene managed the household. She personally maintained the schedules and tasks of our cleaning women and outside support groups. She not only interfaced with the ladies but also became friends with them.

Ilene also disciplined the boys and related to our neighbors when a problem arose. I was seldom called on to perform punishment. The boys respected Mother and her wishes. In all her relationships, Ilene maintained a calm demeanor and would be a caring-but-loving person. This is most remarkable in light of her limited energy and physical limitations.

Personal Maintenance

Ilene was always interested in being able to maintain her appearance and personal dress. Ilene was able to personally perform these functions while at home. Through her rehabilitation, she had become independent so that she could get into and out of bed and use bathroom facilities on her own. She managed our hired help so that they were directed by Ilene to maintain a clean house and to facilitate normal household operations.

This capability meant that our sons and I could be independent of taking care of tasks associated with most nursing functions. Mother had a most normal relationship to us in these matters. It was done so casually that we took it as normal, but it was a major achievement on her part.

Other Roles

Ilene's good cooking and special recipes were well known and appreciated, especially by her children and their friends. It was a tradition that her special homemade birthday cakes were always tailored to the tastes and preferences of the celebrant. This always made a birthday a much-anticipated event. She contributed recipes to the church cookbook. Her dessert specialties were treasured by our son, Jim, who continues to make these desserts to this day.

We happily moved through the years of grade school, high school, college and the marriage of both sons. Anchored in our faith in God and our mutual love, the twenty years from 1980 to 2000 contained many highlights and problems, but always had joy. Our lives were normal, much to the contributions of Ilene.

Here is a photo of Ilene and me at Woodlake Church. Bernt Opsal took the happy picture of us after a Sunday service.

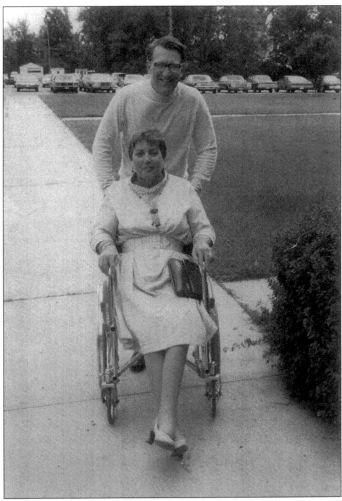

Sunday morning at Woodlake Lutheran Church.

Our relationship to each other grew and resulted in many expressions of love. Two examples:

Ilene's Christmas Revelation: (1983)
The Unmasking of Serge Buskin

We maintained playful communication and were able to see humor in some of the stories of our lives. Most of our talk from the Sheltering Arms period dealt with a new set of words and phrases related to the problems of trying to gain mobility. Sometimes we assumed new identities related to our lives. I had read some of the Russian authors of major works such as Tolstoy, Chekhov, etc.

I maintained jokingly that my true identity was one of a Russian poet, necessarily hidden from the evil Bolsheviks. The Duchy of Finland was most related to czarist Russia from 1809 to WWI. It was, of course, a secret we Finns had to maintain.

> *My dear Serge Bushkin*
>
> *I know who you really are.*
>
> *Your loving, caring and giving spirit has revealed to me that you are really...Jolupuki (Santa Class) I'm so happy to know the real you.*
>
> *Thanks for making Christmas 1993 festive and special.*
>
> *God bless you.*
>
> > *Your everloving,*
> >
> > *Doog, etc.*

My Poem for Ilene's Birthday: (March 7, 1982)

What Shade of Blue?
Blue Eyes
beckoned across Memorial Ballroom
and we began to dance for fun – which continues
Blue Eyes
smiled from a creek in Boone
and started a friendship – which continues
Blue Eyes
brimmed with tears in church
and started a marriage – which continues
Blue Eyes
weakly enters a brown hospital
and left wheeling – which continues
Blue Eyes
peered from an iron lung
and retained courage – which continues
Blue Eyes
closed during Jim's birth
and loved again – which continues
Blue Eyes
view music to sing
and give praise to God – which continues
Blue Eyes
welcome me to a pumpkin house
and give me joy each day – which continues
Blue Eyes
What shade?
Color them Love

This poem is illustrated by the photo of Ilene on the front cover of this book.

Ilene settled into a nearly steady-state physical condition. The doctors at General Hospital had estimated that Ilene's life would be shorted by 18 years. Since Ilene was now about 70 years old and in a fine state of mind and body, we were very joyful for what the Lord had given us. We were, however, in a relatively steady state near the year 2000. We had devised methods of providing maximum mobility. We selected cars with wide doors and leather seats to expedite transfer. With practice and repetition, we had our physical problems "in hand."

Pearl Sorenson was a special friend of Ilene's. She was considered a saint by some. "Saint Pearl" started visiting Ilene when I was on a business trip. Pearl's husband Ed was an airline pilot, so it was an amiable social pairing.

Family

Ruth and Jim established a fine home. Ruth obtained her doctor's degree in nursing from the University of Minnesota and became a professor there. She has won awards for excellence in teaching and was also credited for her research work. Jim became a special agent with the Internal Revenue Service. They have a lovely daughter Rebecca or "Beckie" and a son named Eric. Beckie's name was chosen by her parents, in part, to honor Ilene whose maiden name – Bechtel – was similar. At one time, "Beckie" was also Ilene's nickname.

Ilene and Beckie had a very special relationship, particularly in Beckie's "teenage years." Ilene seemed to understand Beckie and Beckie knew that and appreciated it. Ilene had a special affinity for scarves. Beckie used her great sense of color to pick out a scarf for Ilene's present on most Christmases. When Beckie found the perfect scarf, she would typically exclaim, "This will match Grandma's skin tone and outfits perfectly."

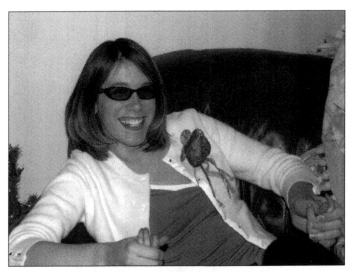

Granddaughter Beckie Lindquist Nguyen.

Grandmother Ilene always prayed for Beckie and this was special to Beckie as well. Beckie still keeps a photo of Grandmother "Peach" in her living room. This is the only family picture Beckie displays.

Tony Nguyen is Beckie's husband and they make a fine team. Tony works a responsible management position for Microsoft. Tony knew Ilene for only a short while but honors her with the picture of Ilene next to his father's picture. His father was a fighter pilot in the Vietnamese Air Force. Tony and Beckie have a well-disciplined, responsive loving family of six children: Jordan, Nicholas, Madison, Isaac, Lyla Peach, and Kane. When Ilene was gravely ill, Beckie mustered her entire family to visit Ilene in the hospital.

As an example of Ilene's influence on Beckie and Tony's family, granddaughter Madison at the age of four was in the middle of the ice rink, dressed in full uniform including hockey skates. She was very upset and in tears with a situation in which she was unable to do what she wanted to do. Madison's grandmother Ruth Ann went out to see what she could do to console her. Madison blurted out, "I miss Grandma Peach!" The essential Ilene had established a loving relationship with little Madison. Perhaps it was because of her readily identifiable wheelchair and her joyful demeanor when she was with her great grandchild.

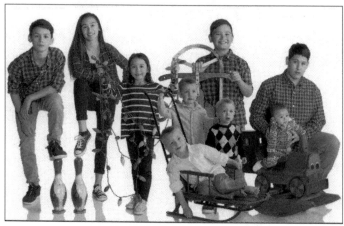

Grandchildren Nicholas, Madison, Lyla Peach, Soren, Liam, Mikkel, Issac, Jordan, and Kane.

Grandson Eric grew into a tall, handsome person who gave us a lot of pleasure in hockey by being on several championship teams and the Gustavus Adolphus College varsity hockey team. These hockey trips to and from St. Peter were joyous occasions for Ilene. The choice of Gustavus also afforded an opportunity for Eric and Marit to get acquainted. This did not happen until their senior year. Since high school, Eric always seemed to have a fine-looking and intelligent girlfriend. He didn't spend much time in pursuit of such a friend as they were the type of girls who took their own initiative in such matters.

Eric was much occupied by doing the best he could at the academic side of school as well as playing hockey – which he did enjoy. Marit states that it took a long time to impress Eric with her merit.

One night during Eric's senior season, we were visited in the stands by Marit's parents, Steve and Debbie Sviggum. We later learned that Steve was the speaker of the House of Representatives in the state legislature.

Eric and Marit were married in the spring of 2009. Ilene was pleased with this arrangement. She had, however, always remained neutral on Eric's girlfriends, although Marit was very special to her. Ilene had a feeling that it would be a great match and that Marit was special.

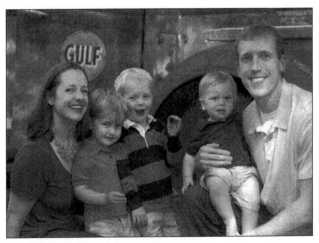

Grandson Eric and wife Marit with sons Liam , Soren and Mikkel.

The advent of grandchildren from Jim's marriage to Ruth expanded our range of activities considerably. A highlight of this part of grandson Eric's career was a national hockey tournament held in Fargo. His team won the tournament and all went well. We had Ruth and Jim to our hotel for supper one night for an enjoyable time. This team was a "squirt" squad that included J.P. Parise's sons. J.P. praised Eric's skating and play and later invited him to attend a private school in Faribault that emphasized hockey. This did not happen because Eric preferred to stay home and play for the Bloomington Jaguars. One of J.P.'s sons has gone on to play in the NHL

My son, Jim, recalls that Ilene had a repertoire of simple instructions on life, some of which may not have always been welcome at the time. As an adult and father of two children of his own, Jim advises that many "Peachisms" were taken off the shelf, dusted off and put into good use in raising his own kids. Jim particularly remembers preferring as a teenager to shroud his out-of-the-home activities in secrecy. When asked for specifics on various outings he planned, his answer was most often, "I don't know." For Ilene, that response did not cut it and her response was always consistently the same, "You had better make it your business to know."

Jim quickly learned that he was not going anywhere until that basic question was answered to Ilene's satisfaction. This expression is one of his favorites with his kids when on many occasions he says, "You know what Grandma Peach used to say"... Jim's kids do not need to hear the full quote; they know it by heart.

Another of Jim's favorites had to do with helping with household work. When in high school, Jim spent hours training for the sports he participated in. In particular, Jim spent a great deal of time lifting weights. Jim recalls one winter when, after a big snowstorm, Ilene asked him to go out and shovel the snow off our driveway. Jim was not too excited about this. It was pretty hard to argue with Ilene's response that was, "You spend so much time lifting weights and exercising for your sports, why don't you spend a little time exercising on our driveway?"

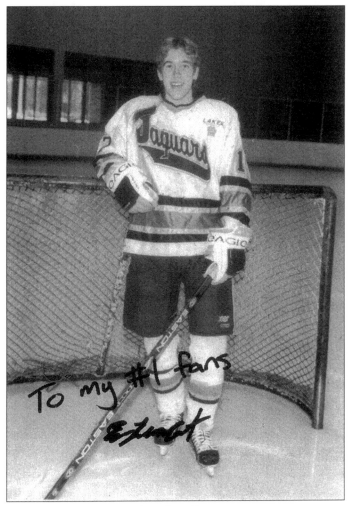

Grandson Eric.

Ilene also had a way of teaching her kids not to be too boastful of their accomplishments. Jim recalls that on one occasion, Ilene had had enough of what she perceived to be Jim's vanity with the muscles he had developed through weight lifting. As a result, one night at the dinner table Ilene threw down the gauntlet and promptly challenged Jim to an arm-wrestling match. Jim sized up the situation and respectfully declined the challenge. He knew his mother had one good arm and that she spent an awful lot of time using it to get around in her wheelchair. To this day, he recalls not being willing to risk the humiliation of defeat against the strong arm of his mother. Lesson learned; humility and respect assured.

CHAPTER 8

2002-2007 – New Problems

Start of the Problem

In 2002, Ilene began to show signs of problems. I noticed that Ilene's stools turned dark – an indication of internal bleeding. After examination by her doctor, and also at Fairview Southdale Hospital, it was determined that she had a stomach cancer that was bleeding. It was of a slow-growing type that had probably been present for some time. She was placed into intensive care before the necessary operation. In this new problem, Ilene retained her calm composure and faced the facts with courage.

It was then determined the bleeding was a result of her taking Advil to help her sleep at night. Advil had not been prescribed, but was not forbidden either. The doctors operated on her and removed the cancer and part of her stomach. Her progress was initially good and she was transferred to a regular private room.

After she was in the private room, she began to have breathing problems and was transferred back to intensive care. Her attending pulmonologist felt that a CPAP oxygen system was adequate, although she might need respiratory aid when she went home. Her primary intensive care nurse had considerable experience with cases such as Ilene's and ordered a ventilator be brought up immediately to assist in breathing. Shortly thereafter, it was decided that a tracheotomy should be performed to further help the problem. This was her second tracheotomy, the first being done while Ilene was breathing with the aid of the iron lung.

At that time, grandson Eric was a sophomore on the Bloomington Jefferson Jaguars high school varsity hockey team. This was quite an achievement as the team had just won the state tournament. He had played on the junior varsity and was also was one of three players frequently invited to sit with the varsity as a "reserve," so he sometimes played on the varsity team. One night Eric visited Ilene at Fairview Hospital just after she had returned to intensive care. Eric was very excited to tell Ilene that the Jaguars were one game away from the annual Minnesota state high school hockey tournament. He had been told that if the team went to the state tournament, that he would be a part of the squad and that he would earn a varsity letter. This was joyous news to Ilene! This was also good news to everyone in the family and it turned out that the Jaguars did go to the state tournament.

The tournament was held in the Excel Energy Center in St. Paul. It is the largest state high school hockey tournament in the USA with a nightly attendance of 18,000. When the teams played their first game in the tournament, all members were individually introduced with full TV coverage. Ilene insisted on being able to watch the tournament on TV. Big Eric skated smartly up to the line and clearly stated while looking at the camera: "Hello, Grandma." We have a prized videotape of that event, even though Eric's team did not win the game.

After we established the news that Ilene was capable of rehabilitation, she was transferred to Bethesda Lutheran Hospital in St. Paul. Ilene progressed well in her breathing and in several weeks she was transferred for a short time to Walker Methodist Health Center. This transfer was for her to regain more function, but it was quickly determined that she would do as well at home.

We employed special nursing services to help us during this rehabilitation period in our transition to home care. Ilene was again not happy to be intruded upon. The total experience was a difficult one for Ilene. She never regained the capabilities that she formerly had.

The stomach operation turned out to result in major problems. The operation resulted in removing a part of Ilene's stomach and prohibited Ilene's previous methods of transfer. A Hoyer Lift and slings were necessary in all transfers to the wheelchair. We also needed a hospital bed at home to accommodate our needs. Ilene was forced to use a bedpan for all of her toilet functions which also necessitated using diapers. Her time away from home was limited to the time the diaper was effective. This restricted us to about a 60-mile radius. We could reach St. Peter for Eric's Gustavus Adolphus College hockey games, but could not travel to Duluth or Ames.

Part of the problem was the marked decrease in Ilene's functions due to post-polio syndrome. Decades after recovering much of their muscular strength, survivors of paralytic polio were reporting unexpected fatigue, pain and weakness. The case appeared to be degeneration of motor neurons. The cause of some of the problems appeared to be precipitated by surgery. In any case, we experienced a physical decline associated with post-polio syndrome.

We purchased a Dodge Caravan that was especially designed for wheelchair occupants. The right seat was removed so that Ilene's wheelchair fit in that space, providing her with a normal outside view.

One of the features of the van was called a "kneeling" which lowered the total incline of the built-in ramp to help with wheelchair entry. We chuckled at the idea of kneeling as we set out before all the church functions at Woodlake. When we arrived at family functions, the great grandchildren would gather around with great interest and anticipation to watch the kneeling of the van.

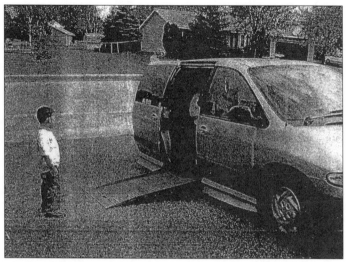

Photo of Beckie's son, Jordan, eagerly awaiting the emergence of "Gramma Peach" before his fifth birthday party.

As time went on, more problems became evident. Ilene had neck problems in holding her head upright. Her strength in her left arm and hand were lost. Ilene maintained a joyful outlook and continued to radiate the Essential Ilene.

> *"But let yours be the hidden person of the heart*
> *with the imperishable jewel of a gentle and*
> *a quiet heart."*
>
> Peter 3:3

We had been traveling to Ames for Ilene's annual high school reunions which were always happy events. The grade-school-through-college friends such as Alice Jean and Wilma would also stay at the motel, providing additional contact.

Throughout her life, Ilene was always impeccably well dressed and well groomed when she left the house. Persons looking at her from the outside had no idea as to how long it took her to prepare herself to go to dinner, to watch the band, or to attend a football or hockey game. She always strove to "look her best" and she did. She was an attractive, well-coiffed and well-dressed woman throughout her life, despite the effort that it took. This "look" was further adorned by her radiant smile.

We did reestablish sufficient mobility to permit attending most events in the cities. The Guthrie and Penumbra Theaters, eating out, visits to local friends and attendance at Jaguars' high school hockey games were again within our range. Grandson Eric's games were especially happy events.

Junior Eric was established as a regular defenseman. Ilene not only enjoyed the games, but also was happy to watch him warm up. He was a very skillful skater and one of the fastest.

During one game, Ilene's dedication to the team was rewarded and formally recognized when she was awarded the pea-green "Jaguar fan of the game" tee shirt by the cheerleaders. The team returned to the state tournament during Eric's senior year.

After high school, Eric wanted to play Division 1 hockey at the University of Minnesota. Coach Don Lucia suggested that he join the Green Bay junior team for a year. The junior hockey system had become the chief source of new players for college Division 1 hockey, with some players playing multiple years before being selected. Eric and family felt that it was too high of a price to pay for only the "potential" for selection. Many MIAC (Minnesota Intercollegiate Athletic Conference) teams were much interested in Eric, but not Division 1 teams. Eric received an invitation to join the University of Connecticut team, which he accepted. The University of Connecticut had an excellent physical therapy program which was of interest to Eric.

Eric spent one year as a "red-shirt" freshman on a losing Connecticut University Division 1 team with a coach he did not enjoy. He decided to return to Minnesota and the MIAC to

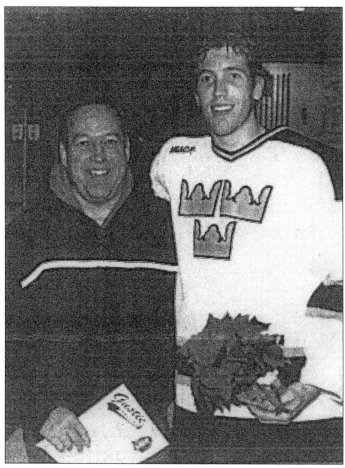

Jim and Eric at a Gustavus home game.

continue his education. He picked Gustavus Adolphus over St. Olaf on the grounds that St. Olaf played on a very inaccessible ice rink for wheelchairs. The "Ole" coach, Coach Goldsworthy ("Goldie"), whose father was a former NHL player (goalie for the North Stars), followed Eric in high school and was most interested in having him play for the Oles. Augsburg had a better facility on campus, but the school did not have appeal to Eric. I arranged a meeting with their coach and also Mark Engelbretson of the physics department to help Eric with his decision.

Gustavus was the best possible choice for Eric and we enjoyed watching Eric play there for three years. Their coach was a mild-mannered, knowledgeable person who gave Eric a major role on the varsity team. The Gustavus ice rink was very accessible to us. There were a small number of stairs to the topside area where we could get the best view of hockey. By careful scheduling of events, we could arrive in St. Peter a few minutes before games, stopping at the local MacDonald's restaurant for burgers and a shake. After the game, we would wait for Eric to come out and we would have a few positive words with him. On the way home, we sometimes ate at Emma Krumbee's Restaurant in Belle Plaine.

Home TV, and especially cable, provided pleasant evening entertainment for Ilene and me. Baseball on TV was superior to going to the dome to watch the game from the remote and isolated handicapped sites.

The restrictions and limits of our lives together began to grow after the 2002 operation for stomach cancer and the tracheotomy. We were able to move to Bethesda Hospital in St. Paul and complete our rehabilitation in about two weeks. Ilene's problem was not her breathing but in recovering from the operation. We had a number of discussions with home rehabilitation services after the operation. They recommended additional home care, which we engaged.

Ilene was not happy with outside service because it was not possible to retain the same person and Ilene was a very private person who preferred her own privacy. The result was that Ilene and I took over more of the household activities. We did, however, begin to have a weekly housekeeper, Phyllis Ford, recommended by a friend who pleased Ilene very much. I engaged a lawn service to reduce my workload. Ilene's problems were also embedded with problems of age and the post-polio syndrome.

We had a hospital bed installed in our bedroom. It was a single bed that could be adjusted to accommodate sitting in bed and adjustable heights. Ilene's reduced capabilities became very apparent during her last year. Her left arm and hand lost strength and she had trouble keeping her head upright. She had also gained weight. When I told her of that problem, she didn't agree with the scale.

The great grandchildren remarked that she seemed to be getting weaker. She also lost some of her ability to eat. We began to take home part of her meals when we ate out.

Ilene was very much aware of her failing capacity. She did maintain a daily devotion that included prayer and Bible study. Her awareness of her problem was reflected in the verses she underlined in the Bible. She did not dwell on her problems, but maintained her faith in God and in the love of Jesus Christ. She knew that God knew her and her problems.

We recognized our need for more help and arranged for home nursing care that was to start the week after we began the last hospital stay. The arrangements were made with a nurse from the nursing agency who noticed Ilene's problem, which seemed like a cold. The nurse warned us that if it started to get worse, we should call 911 immediately. She feared that Ilene had respiratory pneumonia symptoms.

After a few days, Ilene asked me to call 911 because she was having difficulty breathing. I called, and a Richfield medical van arrived. They administered oxygen and suggested that we take Ilene to the Fairview Hospital emergency room immediately, which I did. The four-month end game ensued.

CHAPTER 9

The Second Note – End Game: A Four-Month Struggle

During 2006, several within our family, including great grandchildren, had commented that Peach seemed to be getting weaker. Although her radiance and joy in life continued, her general physical relationships were decreasing. She was content to live her life as fully as possible.

Ilene still was much interested in life and the coming events. Although Eric had finished at Gustavus Adolphus College, he had enrolled in graduate school in a Ph.D. program for physical therapy – a source of great joy. Ilene's role was one of encouragement and prayer.

We always had Friday night out, usually at the Lake Shore Grill at Dayton's Department Store, now Macy's, or some other favorite restaurant such as Lucia's. Ilene continued to have an afternoon devotional that involved Bible study and prayer. We maintained our main church schedule. We required more time to get ready for church. On Sundays, we most generally went to The Good Earth restaurant, usually with friends from our church. The Good Earth staff and some of the regular customers were friendly. Now we had to bring home more leftovers from meals Ilene usually did not finish.

As time went on into 2007, more care for Ilene needed to be done. We were arranging for some additional help at home from Family Home Care. It was scheduled to start on the 12th of July. Ilene was having more difficulty swallowing pills so additional pill pulverizing and swallowing liquids were needed. This became apparent when Ilene had problems swallowing one of her pills. We were making arrangements with nurse Ann Roe from Family Home services. She noticed Ilene's breathing problems and warned us to go to Fairview's emergency room if the conditions grew worse. She anticipated that Ilene might be starting to have symptoms of aspiration pneumonia.

On Thursday, July 5, Ilene began to have breathing difficulty and calmly requested I call 911 and enlist some aid. The Richfield emergency squad arrived and administered oxygen and recovered her oxygen level to an acceptable value. After giving Ilene oxygen, they took her by ambulance to the emergency room at Fairview Southdale Hospital. The final four months of the end game began.

Upon arrival at Fairview Southdale Hospital, Ilene was immediately assigned to intensive care. After examination by the doctors, it was concluded she did have aspiration pneumonia and she had additional problems as well. Lung x-rays revealed additional shadows on her lungs indicating a failure in the respiration process. The Fairview doctors, familiar with her prior hospitalization expressed amazement that she had lived so long, and warned that recovery from the current condition would be more difficult. They were not optimistic of her being able to recover enough to resume independent living. The oxygen-blood exchange was insufficient for a person in her condition.

Despite this information, Ilene felt she could recover and did everything in her power to do so. She was willing to undergo all medical procedures and to make a best-effort attempt to gain freedom for independent living. A ventilator was immediately ordered to help her breathing. The ventilator could provide additional oxygen as well as ventilation assistance. Ilene's heartbeat was low (in the 40s with between 60 and 100 being normal), so drugs were administered to bring it to normal. Some of the attending doctors concluded she was a candidate for a pacemaker. Specialists from the heart clinic were consulted and they felt her heart would not benefit from a pacemaker. The issue at Fairview was to stabilize her and then determine if she could be brought to a condition for a rehabilitation center, or whether she would need a more intensive care center.

During her time at the hospital, Ilene became the godmother of her first great-grandchild, Jordan Manuel. (Eric was the godfather.) She was unable to attend the baptism held at the Community of the Cross church because she was hospitalized, but she constantly prayed for Jordan and all of her family. Her earnest prayers have been a blessing to us all.

Tests and an examination identified the problems Ilene was facing. In addition to her breathing difficulties, the question of her heart function was again brought up. On the evening of July 22, her pulse dropped to 30. The doctors now agreed that a pacemaker should be implanted. Ilene's personal physician felt that the pacemaker was absolutely needed. Further tests included an electrocardiogram (EKG). When we returned to intensive care, it was concluded she needed a pacemaker before she could be rehabilitated. The operation was performed on July 23 and took 45 minutes.

Similar reasoning applied to a tracheotomy operation that was performed. It was needed to permit Ilene's progress toward becoming a candidate for rehabilitation at Bethesda Lutheran Hospital, where she had been treated in 2000 after an operation for stomach cancer.

Following the two operations, Ilene improved and x-rays of her lungs showed lung improvement. She was able to have satisfactory heartbeats without medicine. She was able to breathe without ventilator assistance for up to eight hours on several days. The lead physician, Dr. Stang, stated she was ready for transfer.

She became a candidate for transfer to the Bethesda Lutheran Rehabilitation Hospital in St. Paul on July 27, and transferred the following Monday, July 30. This was a major milestone that gave hope to being able to duplicate our 2000 experience. She was transferred by ambulance to Bethesda at 4:30 on July 30.

At Bethesda Hospital

Dr. Scanlon was the in-charge physician at Bethesda who had also been with Ilene in 2000. Nurse Sandy Carson, who helped admit Ilene, predicted that 25 to 30 days would be required at Bethesda. However, Dr. Scanlon again warned that the current situation was not like her 2000 situation. The quarters at the hospital were much improved. Based upon discussions at Fairview, Ilene wrote a note that the facility was air conditioned. Transfer to Bethesda implied the acute problems were over and rehabilitation could be started.

One of the visits by the family to Bethesda was made on Eric's birthday, August third. He visited with Ilene along with his parents Jim and Ruth. An unexpected surprise was when their daughter, Beckie and her husband Tony came with their sons Jordan and baby Isaac. Tony commented on how pleased Ilene seemed to be to see her godson and baby Isaac. After the visit, the family said a loving good night to Ilene and then went to Mia Village Restaurant where they were joined by Marit Sviggum for dinner in honor of Eric's birthday.

Later, a crisis occurred one evening when Ilene stopped breathing for some unknown cause. The condition was quickly improved by a bevy of people including the therapist Sam. It was later reported that the problem was caused by phlegm blocking her tracheotomy. The problem set Ilene back about a week as she was fed intravenously and no attempts at independent breathing were made.

Ilene's first breathing without a ventilator did not occur until August 6. She continued on this routine until Monday, August 12, when she was increased to four-hour intervals. She also began to have food by mouth on August 6. Her time off the ventilator remained limited. During this time, Ilene made it clear she did not want emergency cardiopulmonary resuscitation, or any extreme measures used on her. She anticipated that not all was going well and did not want unusual procedures used to prolong her life. She had this information attached to her wristband. Ilene was not interested in being in another facility.

The setback was difficult. Bethesda was not an intensive-care hospital and had limited facilities in such matters. In addition, she continued to require antibiotics for infections that were associated with her tracheotomy. On August 31, Dr. Scanlon stated that her blood tests suggested a problem. These were conducted at adjacent St. Joseph's Hospital.

The results were not told to me. By September 6, Ilene had reached 8.5 hours off the ventilator. The rehabilitation team, including Dr. Scanlon, felt Ilene had reached a plateau and that we should start planning for a transfer to another facility.

In anticipation of a return to home, on September 7, I talked to nurse Ann Roe about what could be done in making a transfer to home. She stated that Home Watch did not provide ventilator care and that a 24-hour nurse would be required. This situation would therefore seem to demand some type of facility capable of intensive care.

I reviewed the situation with Ilene after these meetings. She calmly accepted the information, and she immediately began making efforts to improve her condition. The next day she breathed 11.5 hours without the ventilator and began taking meals in her chair. She also increased her time with a speech valve to 6.5 hours. It was more difficult to breath with a speech valve in place. She continued to show improvement and was able to spend half days without ventilator help. The rehabilitation team noticed the positive improvement and was impressed with her courage and the progress that she seemed to will.

Ilene was increasing the time out of bed and in a wheelchair. The rehab team then planned to start capping off the trach and having all breathing via normal channels. This was the most positive time of the Bethesda experience. Her efforts brought new progress and generated new hope.

The team also inserted a new smaller tracheotomy tube. On September 14, Ilene breathed 11 hours off the ventilator and one hour with the trach tube covered. Covering the trach tube forced her to breath totally on her own via her own airway track. The next day she again did 14 hours using the trach tube without a ventilator, but only 15 minutes with the trach covered.

This presented a new problem. Dr. Wright, the respiratory doctor, talked to Ilene and me on September 20 regarding the problem of breathing with the trach capped off. The negative pressure in the trach tube was closing the passageway above the tracheotomy tube. He decided to prescribe steroids (Prednisone) for a week to reduce inflammation and cure the problem of the trach tube. He said that if this did not cure the problem, they would use laser surgery to enlarge the passage. If this didn't help, Ilene would have to keep the trach tube.

Dr. Latham thought Ilene was doing better. She was able to breathe without the ventilator for several hours every day. Grandson Eric visited for one-and-a-half hours on September 21. It was a very fine visit. Eric and I ate lunch in the gazebo.

On October 4, Dr. Wright stated an operation would be scheduled to take off inflamed tissue above the trach tube. This procedure was crucial to being able to breathe without a ventilator. At that meeting, Ilene again stated she did not want resuscitation or unusual procedures.

Pastor Mark Wegener gave Ilene communion on October 5. Dr. Kristen Gendron, the surgeon for the operation, came in to discuss the operation. She gave Ilene a preview of the operation. She stated that the operation was sometimes done on an outpatient procedure. She stated she would not use laser in this operation. The operation was scheduled for Thursday, October 10 at St. Joseph's Hospital at 7:30 a.m.

Our neighbors, Vern and Dorothy Lace, visited on October 8. It was a very happy interchange. Ilene was talking via a voice box on CPAc.

At 6:30 a.m. on October 11, Ilene was transported to St. Joseph's Hospital. The two-and-a-half-hour operation was performed. Afterwards, Dr. Gendron stated that there was only a 50-50 chance that the trach could be removed and that there would be a problem trying to reinsert a new one.

On October 14, Ilene had an infection and an antibiotic was started. Problems developed keeping the IV flowing and this problem continued.

The attempt to cover the trach on October 17 lasted two hours. A second attempt on October 18 was stopped after one hour. Ilene was having breathing problems and requested aid. Covering the trach was stopped. On October 19, Dr. Gendron visited and said the problems were not caused by the operation.

Reverend Wegener visited briefly. Lung x-rays and blood tests were OK. Ilene rested all day. On October 20, Ilene was tired and having breathing difficulty.

On Sunday, October 21, I received a call from a nurse at Bethesda at 4:30 a.m. Ilene wanted me to come. I arrived at 6 and found that Ilene was having extreme breathing problems. The technicians had already increased the ventilator pressure and percent of oxygen. Ilene had managed to write the second note for me.

Note: October 21, 2007

(Bethesda Hospital, St. Paul)
I spent all night struggling to breathe.
It has been a fight to go on.
I don't want to struggle any more.
I'm ready to go.
My wristband says I don't want
extreme measures. I can't even eat.
I want to be taken off respirator.
Please.

The respiratory therapists were forced to increase the percentage of oxygen used with the ventilator. This was a major problem and they called for help. The medical staff took action to determine the problem. They took chest x-rays and the electrocardiograph indicated Ilene was having atrial fibrillation. Dr. Black of the hospital staff stated that Ilene would have to be transferred to a hospital better able to handle the crisis. I suggested Fairview Southdale, and Ilene was immediately transferred by ambulance on Sunday, October 21.

Return to Fairview Southdale Emergency

The emergency medical team informed us that Ilene's problem was acute and that her blood pressure was 60/40 which was not enough to support life. The doctors administered a drug to increase blood pressure which was successful so that Ilene could be moved to intensive care.

Visits were made by Dan, Jim, Ruth, Beckie. Tony and Eric. Beckie visited her beloved grandmother several times with Tony during this hospitalization.

On October 21, Ilene responded to treatment but was still considered in critical condition. She was transferred to intensive care. She had to be on the ventilator with nearly 100% oxygen, an undesirable condition.

On October 23, Dr. Steele informed us that Ilene was still critical and we were in extreme measures. Reverend Diane Roth visited but was not able to give communion.

Jim, Dan, Ruth and I held a 6:30 family meeting. We reviewed the condition and the problems. We also reviewed Note Two. We all knew the situation. We felt we should wait for possible improvement (days) and then determine the possible outcomes when we would then consider the reasonable course of action.

On October 24, it was determined that the implanted trach tube was the problem and that it had either failed or was defective. The tube was replaced with a temporary tube until a new tube could be found. When I arrived in the morning, hospital staff was using x-rays to help position the tube. Ilene continued to experience atrial fibrillation. By noon, the situation was stable, and her blood pressure was 100/50. A discussion with Dr. Bohlen indicated the lung problems were increasing. He felt that the two months of progress at Bethesda were lost and that Ilene would have to go through that experience again.

On October 25, Dr. Mellon of Fairview Southdale Hospital advised that it was time to let Ilene go. He recommended that we inform Ilene of the situation. A new trach tube had arrived. Dr. Bohlen agreed with Dr. Mellon.

On October 26, Dr. Stang stated that it was taking heavy pressure and 100% oxygen to keep Ilene going. He felt it would take a long time to become less dependent upon a ventilator and that she may not get better at all. We asked the social worker, Sandy Duetech, to set up a Monday meeting at 9:30 to review Ilene's case with the family.

We had a visit from Jim, Dan, Marit, Eric and Ruth. Ilene worked hard to stay with the group, but faded out. Eric kissed and hugged Peach. Ilene seemed to "hang in there," committed to her faith and her family, especially, it seemed, for me. Dan sat with his mother often. She took great comfort in this. One night, when Jim was sitting alone with Ilene in the intensive care unit, Jim told her that if she lost this fight that he would take care of his father. She nodded and mouthed the words, "I know you will."

After four months at Fairview and Bethesda hospitals, Ilene's problems were severe in her mind. She had done everything they had asked her to do, and the yet situation seemed back to square one. The doctors had initiated the last operation to facilitate weaning from the tracheotomy, a necessary step enabling a return to home. The care and tendency for infection were said to be the cause for transfer to another institution of some type. It had obviously failed and her problems were acute and severe.

Ilene's faith in the Lord Jesus Christ who loved her did not require her to struggle toward an unknown end that would not be satisfactory. She had already stated she did not want unusual measures taken in her life. She had done her best and she felt it was time to go home to God. She had been reduced in function to only being able to move her right arm, and from the handwriting in her note, her physical weakness was obvious, but her will was clear.

Her care and feeding prior to hospitalization while at home was already difficult, and although we had just finished arranging for more health care, the agency would not handle a ventilator patient like Ilene at home. Her reference to not even being able to eat was a reference to our many evenings out, especially the Sunday after-church brunches at The Good Earth at the Galleria in Edina. She had already been having trouble eating before the last episode began. She was effectively saying she foresaw a dismal future that was not necessary. She had done her best, even enjoying even the last four months, but this was enough. There was no task left for her to do, She faced these facts courageously.

The final "Please" was a direct request to me. I don't remember having her ever ask for anything like that. I knew it was my turn to act.

I still needed to gather the facts and obtain agreement from the family – but a final decision and action was required.

October 27. The new trach failed again. Dr. Bohlen felt there was scar tissue that tore the mechanism. He stated that they were forced to use maximum ventilator pressure and 100% oxygen, and this condition meant Ilene could not survive until Monday. She would probably not regain consciousness and that no other treatment was possible. We were only prolonging death.

Jim, Dan and I all agreed – let her go. I monitored the final act. She was taken off the ventilator and quickly and quietly she died.

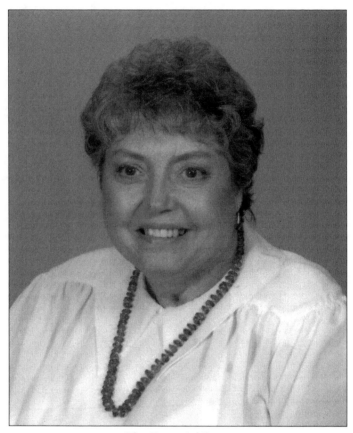

The Essential Ilene.

Epilogue

In chess, the pawn moves slowly initially and is the most restricted piece on a chessboard. It is the piece that is most limited in action, but can be later transformed to a queen. Polio had restricted Ilene to a wheelchair and finally to very limited, slow actions. Ilene is now transformed to a Queen because she is at home with a loving Jesus.

She spent over two years of her life in hospitals. Her restrictions and problems included being alone in hospitals at night with uncertainty as to what was coming next. She knew in faith that she was known and loved by God. She expressed this faith as best as she could whenever possible. The "Essential Ilene" was a most responsive person in relationships and she always conveyed love.

Her funeral service was held on November 2, 2007, with our minister, Dr. Mark Wegener, presiding. A moving eulogy was given by Reverend Jack Bredfeldt, a long-time Christian friend who was an usher at our wedding and a missionary to Africa for a number of years.

After Ilene's death, a note was received from the doctor who was in charge of her case at Bethesda Lutheran hospital both in 2000 and in 2007. Dr. Scanlon wrote the note with regard to his experience with Ilene.

November 7, 2007

Dear Herb and family of Ruth,

We were sorry to hear of Ruth's death at Fairview. We did our best to help her at Bethesda but her pulmonary problem became too severe. I and all who cared for Ruth admired her tenacity and will to live, despite great and overwhelming illness, she always maintained a pleasant, dignified and positive outlook.

I received a great outpouring of condolences, prayers and love from many friends. One touching contact was from a former Sunday school pupil of Ilene's at Grace Lutheran in Bloomington. Ilene was told by Reverend Christianson of a young girl's problems related to her mother's suicide. Ilene had worked to help her in every way she could. This woman called me from Chicago to express her condolences to me. She wanted to know if Ilene was aware of her personal problems when they had been in contact at Grace. She started crying on the phone for an hour and a half as we talked. She had become a counselor herself as a profession.

Ilene never gave up until there was no hope for her being in anything but an institution with extensive care facilities. She underlined the following in her Bible:

> *For to me to live is Christ, and to die is gain. If it*
> *is to be life in the flesh, that means fruitful labor*
> *for me. Yet which I choose I cannot tell. I am hard*
> *pressed between the two. My desire is to depart*
> *and be with Christ, for that is far better.*
> *Philippines 1:21*

Ilene had reached the point where she could not envision her fruitful labor and she wanted to be with her Savior Jesus Christ. She was secure in her faith and in courage.

Ilene spent a great deal of time and thought in giving her annual talk to the Stephen Ministry of Woodlake Lutheran Church. The Stephan Ministry was a visitation program to homebound. This was a unique speech by an individual who considered this ministry a major element in their life. She considered this speech a mission of her life. The words from her word processor indicate the content of her speech.

These words were totally her own and she worked hard to make them personal and relevant. Her speech was a culmination of years of effort first started by a request from the Reverend Robert Hall of our church. Ilene's address was well received by the group and was an inspiration to many of them. A physically handicapped woman in a wheelchair – with a loving, accepting spirit who obviously enjoyed life, and worshiped God – was an impelling speaker. She wanted to contribute to someone else. This was exactly the thrust of the Stephen Ministry program.

Ilene's Stephen Ministry Speech concludes this book. THer speech is a transparent look at the honest nature of her faith and view of life. She was regularly asked to address the Stephen ministers at our church. She spent a great deal of time and effort to make her vows clearly known. Beyond the thoughts in her paper, it was delivered by a person with a bright life who was capable of loving; who enjoyed people and life. We had the text copied and passed it out at Ilene's funeral.

This book was written to help understand the "Essential Ilene," a Christian woman of great courage and love for family, and of great faith and love for her Lord and Savior Jesus Christ.

Stephen Ministry Presentation

Presented by Ilene Lindquist on May 20, 2003, to the Stephen Ministers at Woodlake Lutheran Church in Richfield, Minnesota.

> *I know the plans I have for you, says the Lord, plans*
> *for welfare and not for eveil, to give you a future and*
> *a hope. Then you will call upon me and come to pray*
> *to me, and I will hear you.*
> Jeremiah 29: 11-12

> *Behold I have graven you on the palms of my hands.*
> Isaiah 49:16

The living God says to me He wants a relationship with me and He has plans for my welfare and future. He has a hope for me. He know me intimately because He has written me on the palms of His hands.

I have the hope He speaks of for this life and for eternal life through faith in the gospel of Jesus Christ. We have just recently celebrated the resurrection of Christ. Some of you may recall that Woodlake gave some support to Pastor John Melin when he served as pastor in an ecumenical church in Moscow. We received a copy of his Easter sermon one year. In it he said something I would like to quote because I think it speaks to what I have been saying. "Easter proclaims that there is nothing final in suffering and death. The future is open; there is more to come. Christ has conquered all that seeks to conquer us. To believe in a creating and recreating God is to trust the possibilities of life and to know that what will be is more and better than what has been."

The lifetime relationship that I have had with God is the most important one in my life. I see all other relationships through it. Christ has made peace with God for me; He has paid the price for my sin. When in faith I believe this, I have God's peace with me and am able to reach out to my neighbor with the love of God.

> *Bear ye one another's burdens and so fulfill the law of Christ.*
> Galatians 6:2

You as Stephen Ministers can be a caring friend to someone who is hurting and needs you to be there for them. Another way that my faith in Christ helps me is the issue of identity and self worth. I'm sure that as you minister, you find those with difficulty accepting who they are. Here is an example to think about.

The world-famed cellist Yo Yo Ma was being interviewed by Charlie Rose on TV. Rose said to him, "You were born in Paris of Chinese parents. You studied at Harvard and the Juilliard School of Music, and you play with orchestras in all capitals of the world. How do you think of yourself: Chinese, French musician, or what? Yo Yo Ma replied, "Well, I'm *me*."

This is how I feel about myself; my identity. It seems to me that we cannot view our identity or derive our self worth from being a member of a particular group, be it black, disabled, senior, woman, etc. The reality of my life is that I am disabled. But the essential "me" is much more than that. I want people to know *me*. I have interests and abilities that have nothing to do with my disability.

One of the questions I have most frequently been asked is whether I can walk or will ever be able to. Being able to walk is surely very important, especially to a formerly physically active person, but life can be lived fully without this ability. I can only know who I am through a relationship with Jesus Christ. My self worth comes from the value God has placed on my life. Through faith, I know that Christ has loved me so much that He has given His life for me. In thankfulness to Him, I have chosen to live the life He has given me through faith in Christ to glorify Him with it. I accept the hard times as well as the good.

*When you pass thru the waters, I will be with you;
and thru the rivers, they shall not overwhelm you;
when you walk thru fire you shall not be burned, and
the flame shall not consume you. For I am the Lord
your God.*
Isaiah 3:3

What a promise God has given that as we go through life with
its various circumstances and difficulties, He will be there with us.
I have experienced His presence in my life, helping me to accept
and deal with difficulties even though He may not move them.

As I said at the beginning, I believe God has plans for my life
now and for eternity. Within the frame of time, events, relationships and circumstances that God has given me, I have chosen
to live by faith in Christ.

About the Author

Oiva Herbert (Herb) Lindquist is the only child of Karl Lindquist and Hannah Ahro Lindquist. Herb grew up in the woods and lakes of northern Minnesota where he fished, explored and enjoyed academics and athletics.

After serving in the Army and as a naval cadet during World War II, Herb earned a bachelor's degree in physics at Iowa State University where he met and married his late wife, Ilene. When Ilene contracted polio in 1952, Herb left teaching physics at Augsburg College and began his 32-year career at Honeywell, Inc. Herb founded Augsburg's physics department and is still involved with developing the department. Herb and Ilene have two sons.

Space Engineering Manager, Honeywell, Inc.

With a masters degree in biophysics from the University of Minnesota, Herb became the space engineering manager at Honeywell, initiating man-machine system analysis and development. This capability resulted in numerous products and participation in advanced-systems development including space projects such as the space station and several aircraft programs.

Apollo Moon Project

For more than five years, Herb participated in studies to define astronauts' mission role and their display-control interface with equipment. Upon being awarded the contract to North American in Downy, California, Honeywell was selected as Stabilization Control System Provider. Herb became the section head of the systems group that analyzed, designed and released specifications for construction of equipment used on all Apollo spacecraft flights. This included flight-director attitude display, hand controllers, autopilot and control electronics.

Made in the USA
Coppell, TX
28 December 2023

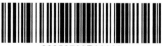

26953700R00068